ON-CALL
in Oral and Maxillofacial Surgery

Karl F.B. Payne
Clinical Fellow in Oral and Maxillofacial Surgery
King's College Hospital, London, UK

Alexander M.C. Goodson
Clinical Fellow in Oral and Maxillofacial Surgery
King's College Hospital, London, UK

Arpan S. Tahim
Clinical Fellow in Oral and Maxillofacial Surgery
King's College Hospital, London, UK

Nabeela Ahmed
Specialty Trainee in Oral and Maxillofacial Surgery
King's College Hospital, London, UK

Kathleen Fan
Consultant Oral and Maxillofacial Surgeon
King's College Hospital, London, UK

Foreword by:
Professor Mark McGurk
Professor of Oral and Maxillofacial Surgery
Guy's Hospital, London, UK

Photographs by:
Margaret Delaney-Quirke RMIP
Senior Medical Photographer
King's College Hospital, London, UK

First published in 2014 by Libri Publishing

Copyright © Karl F.B. Payne, Alexander M.C. Goodson, Arpan Tahim, Nabeela Ahmed and Kathleen Fan

The right of Karl F.B. Payne, Alexander M.C. Goodson, Arpan Tahim, Nabeela Ahmed and Kathleen Fan to be identified as the authors of this work has been asserted in accordance with the Copyright, Designs and Patents Act, 1988.

ISBN 978 1 909818 15 6

All rights reserved. No part of this publication may be reproduced, stored in any retrieval system or transmitted in any form or by any means, electronic, mechanical, photocopying, recording or otherwise, without the prior written permission of the copyright holder for which application should be addressed in the first instance to the publishers. No liability shall be attached to the author, the copyright holder or the publishers for loss or damage of any nature suffered as a result of reliance on the reproduction of any of the contents of this publication or any errors or omissions in its contents.

A CIP catalogue record for this book is available from The British Library

Cover and Design by Carnegie Publishing

Printed in the UK by Berforts Information Press

Libri Publishing
Brunel House
Volunteer Way
Faringdon
Oxfordshire
SN7 7YR

Tel: +44 (0)845 873 3837

www.libripublishing.co.uk

CONTENTS

Dedication — iv
Abbreviations — v
Foreword — vii
Introduction — 1
Disclaimer — 2

Essentials — 3

Referrals — 3
Ward administration — 5
Admission clerking for elective and emergency patients — 7
An introduction to teeth — 12
Dental occlusion — 17
Anatomy — 19
Radiology — 32
Drugs — 37
Oral surgery instruments — 39

Emergency Department — 41

Assessment and initial management of facial trauma — 41
Midfacial fractures — 48
Mandibular fractures — 55
Retrobulbar haemorrhage (RBH) – acute orbital compartment syndrome — 57
Head injuries — 59
Facial lacerations — 61
Facial burns — 65
Epistaxis — 67
Post extraction complications — 69
Dental trauma — 72
TMJ dislocation — 75
Orofacial and neck space infections — 77

Ludwig's angina	82
Acute sialadenitis	83
Infected sebaceous cyst	84
Penetrating neck injury	85
Bleeding and ulcerated gums	87

Ward — 89

Prescribing intravenous fluids	89
Patients with altered fluid/electrolyte requirements	91
Glucose control	94
Tracheostomies	97
Flaps in oral and maxillofacial reconstruction	100
Enteral feeding	103
Evaluating the acutely 'unwell' patient	106
Patients on warfarin	109

Clinic — 111

Acute trauma clinic	111
Oncology clinic	115
Salivary gland clinic	119
Facial skin lesions	122
Oral soft tissue lesions	125
Suspected oral malignancy	131
TMJ presentations	133
Trigeminal neuralgia	136
Facial and oral pain	136
Pre-operative assessment clinic	138
Consenting a patient for surgery	142
Benefits and risks of specific surgical procedures	144
Post-operative review clinic	151

Procedures　　　　　　　　　　　　　　　　**155**

Venepuncture, IV cannulation and taking blood cultures	155
Nerve blocks of the mouth and face	160
Tooth splinting	170
Suturing of the face and mouth	173
Bridle wiring	178
Nasal packing	180
Draining abscesses under local anaesthetic	184
Pinna haematoma	186
Septal haematoma	188
Flexible nasoendoscopy	189
Lateral canthotomy	192

Index　　　　　　　　　　　　　　　　　　194

DEDICATION

This book is dedicated to Caroline, Claire, Susan, Adam and Tim, for their patience throughout multiple university degrees and continued perseverance during the ever-continuing training in maxillofacial surgery!

We acknowledge Miss Elinor Carey for kindly volunteering to model within this book.

ABBREVIATIONS

CN – Cranial nerve
CSF – Cerebrospinal fluid
CT – Computed Tomography
DPT – Dental Panoramic Tomogram (analogous to OPG)
ED – Emergency Department
ENT – Ear Nose and Throat (surgery)
FOM – Floor of mouth
GA – General anaesthetic
GDP – General Dental Practitioner
GP – General (Medical) Practitioner
IM – Intramuscular
IMF – Intermaxillary fixation
IV – Intravenous
LA – Local anaesthetic
MIO – Maximum incisal opening
NBM – Nil by Mouth
NSAID – Non-steroidal anti-inflammatory drug
OMF – Oral and Maxillofacial
OMFS – Oral and Maxillofacial Surgery
OPG – Orthopantomogram (analogous to DPT)
PA – Posteroanterior
PO – Per os (by mouth or orally)
RBH – Retrobulbar haemorrhage
ROS – Removal of sutures
SALT – Speech and Language Therapy
SC – Subcutaneous
SCM – Sternocleidomastoid (muscle)
TMJ – Temporomandibular joint
VTE – Venous Thromboembolism

FOREWORD

This book is timely and fills a real void in clinical practice. The disintegration of the "Firm" structure with the substitution of a shift system in the modern health service has meant that there is a continual rotation of junior staff with little knowledge of or exposure to Oral and Maxillofacial Surgery. This is compounded by the fact that in Maxillofacial Surgery, junior posts are manned by a mixture of dental or medically trained staff who are then exposed to both dental and medical conditions with which they may not be fully familiar. This book ably fills the knowledge gap for both these groups. The book is well written and its great value is that the content has been developed by young Maxillofacial Surgeons during their training, and then refined and polished under the eye of K Fan, a consultant Oral and Maxillofacial Surgeon at Kings College Hospital, London. The content of each chapter arises from problems that they have experienced and the knowledge conferred fits perfectly the needs of the on-call junior surgeon faced with the responsibility for the Oral and Maxillofacial service. This book is a tribute to the authors for its worth extends far outside its target audience and contains important information for Emergency clinicians and those managing Head and Neck oncology wards. A copy of this book should be on every Oral and Maxillofacial ward and in every hospital's Emergency Department. It is essential reading for junior surgeons who in their training are precipitously exposed to patients presenting with disorders in the Head and Neck.

Professor Mark McGurk

INTRODUCTION

Oral and Maxillofacial Surgery is the specialty which manages acute and chronic disorders of the face, neck, mouth and jaws. Because this anatomical region is highly complex, OMF surgeons must be trained in managing a wide variety of presentations with many different surgical techniques. Trainees in OMFS must have a good grasp of face and neck trauma, orofacial and neck-space infections, head & neck oncology, elective head & neck reconstruction including free-tissue transfer, orthognathic treatment, benign conditions of the skin and oral cavity, dento-alveolar disease and aesthetic facial surgery. Because of the vast array of conditions managed by OMF surgeons, internationally the majority are dual-qualified in both medicine and dentistry, using skills drawn from both fields. However, as the 'first-on-call' clinician, the average newcomer to the specialty is typically singly-qualified in either medicine or dentistry, leaving the potential for a significant knowledge gap when attempting to manage OMFS presentations. This can be a daunting prospect for any junior (as the authors are well aware!), and for this reason, *On-call in Oral and Maxillofacial Surgery* was born.

This book aims to give the junior OMF surgeon an introductory grasp of the specialty. Using it as a 'survival guide' the reader will learn how to take emergency referrals for patients from the ED, and institute initial management of common OMFS presentations before recruiting the help of a senior. The reader will also learn about day-to-day management of inpatients on the ward, as well as dealing with patients in the clinic environment. Finally, practical step-by-step guidance is provided for minor surgical procedures, often performed by the junior OMF surgeon.

This book will serve you well if read prior to starting your first job in OMFS, but will also remain a valuable resource on a day-to-day basis as a concise, quick-reference text. We hope that you find this book as useful and interesting as we did writing it.

KP

AG

AT

NA

KF

DISCLAIMER

This book is not a textbook, but a survival guide. All content has been written by the authors and is obtained from reliable sources and based on personal experience. The authors and publisher do not accept responsibility or legal liability for injury or damage to any person as a result of action or refraining from action due to the clinical material within this book. At the time of printing drug doses contained within this book were correct, but it is the reader's responsibility to check up-to-date manufacture and drug dose safety guidelines.

ESSENTIALS

REFERRALS

When on-call in OMFS you will take referrals either from within your institute (typically from the ED or inpatient wards) or from outside the hospital (namely GDPs, GPs or other hospitals). While it is useful to develop a standardised approach to referrals, there are several points to consider depending upon the referring clinician.

GENERAL PRINCIPLES

It is essential to accurately record the referrals you receive:

- Note the time and date when you received the referral.
- Get a brief but full history from the referring clinician, to include: mechanism and time of injury, age of patient, any relevant co-morbidities, etc.
- Document the referring clinicians' name, grade and bleep/extension number.
- Note time since last meal in case the patient requires a GA.

ED REFERRALS

- Make sure the disease or injury falls into the remit of your department i.e. should the patient be referred to a different team? Some patients may need to be admitted with care under two teams – 'joint care'. You will likely need to discuss this with your on-call senior.
- In cases of trauma, always ask about head injury status and whether the cervical spine has been cleared. This should usually be assessed, managed and cleared by the ED team. Remember approximately 1 in 5 OMFS trauma cases are associated with a cervical spine injury.
- Don't be afraid to stand your ground and ask for time to consult a senior colleague before agreeing to see a patient or accept them under your team's care.
- When documenting your notes, be precise about when you were referred the patient and when you assessed them.

WARD REFERRALS

- Do they need to be seen by the OMFS department?
- Is this patient going to need an urgent senior review? If so discuss with your on-call senior.
- It is reasonable to ask for investigations to be organised by the referring team, so you have the results when you formally assess the patient, i.e. a radiograph or blood tests.

GDP AND GP REFERRALS

- Does the patient need to be seen immediately or can they be appropriately seen in the outpatient clinic? If so, be sure to document the patient's full name, address and contact number.
- Depending on your department protocol, you may need to ask for a faxed referral.

HOSPITAL REFERRALS

In addition to the above:

- What time is the patient being referred? Is it appropriate for the patient to travel in the middle of the night? Lacerations in children/adults may be able to wait till the morning if there is no acute bleeding or suspicion of other serious injuries.
- Is the patient fit to be transferred? Are there any airway concerns?
- Observations for head injury should be dealt with at the referring unit before the patient is transferred for non-emergency maxillofacial treatment.
- If you are accepting a patient you will need to speak to your bed manager and see if there is a vacant surgical bed.
- Is the patient going to theatre, hence should they be NBM?
- Clinicians from other hospitals will often be in a rush and may pressure you to make a decision. Be aware of important questions to ask relating to different presentations, e.g. eye signs in orbital fractures, or trismus in dental infections. On this occasion getting a thorough history over the phone is mandatory, to help you or a senior decide upon the best course of action.

Needless to say, if you are in doubt about a referral or whether to accept a patient then always consult your on-call senior. As you gain more experience referrals will become routine, but early on in your first job there is no shame in asking for help.

WARD ADMINISTRATION

STRUCTURING AN INPATIENT LIST

Most OMFS departments will have a computerised, ongoing, day-to-day inpatient list. This list should have details of all inpatients and elective/emergency patients in theatre. The gold standard is a computerised database, but a simple tabulated text document will also suffice. While each department will have its own preferences, the list below covers most of the points that should be recorded for each patient on an inpatient list.

- Name and hospital number
- Age and date of birth
- Date of admission
- Treatment group i.e. emergency, elective, pre-op, post-op
- Diagnosis
- Current problem
- Task list

ADMITTING A PATIENT FROM THE ED

If you are admitting your patient it is usually necessary to:

- Inform the hospital bed manager
- Appropriately consent the patient for the relevant operative procedure
- If an urgent procedure is required, liaise with the on-call anaesthetist and operating department manager before booking the patient onto the emergency operating list.

Prescribe the patient's regular medications and the following:

- VTE prophylaxis according to your hospital protocol
- Analgesia (as required)
- Antiemetics (if required)
- IV fluids
- Antibiotics (if required)

DISCHARGE SUMMARY

The discharge summary is a succinct record of the entirety of the patient's recent hospital stay. It is written primarily for the patient's GP, but can also be of great benefit to a hospital doctor at future admissions where it can provide a useful summary of the patient's past medical history and previous admissions.

Classically these documents were hand-written by junior doctors, often illegibly. To improve standards the majority of hospitals now utilise an electronic discharge summary/document (EDS/EDD). Although these may vary from hospital to hospital, the basic structure and content is the same.

CHECKLIST:
- Are the patient details/sticker correct? Don't write a summary for the wrong patient!
- Date patient was admitted, and under which team
- Presenting complaint, symptoms and diagnosis
- Past medical history
- Investigations ordered and the relevant findings
- Details of management i.e. medications given, etc.
- If underwent surgery: exact procedure performed, details of procedure if required, success of procedure, any complications, post-op instructions
- Full list of all medications when the patient was admitted
- Any omissions or additions to medications
- Follow-up appointment
- Specific instructions to GP with regards to further management

ADMISSION CLERKING FOR ELECTIVE AND EMERGENCY PATIENTS

The following describes the process of undertaking a full history and examination, i.e. 'clerking in' a patient. It can be applied to pre-operative clerking of elective procedure patients (see 'Pre-operative Assessment Clinic' page 138) or emergency admissions (via the ED). Individual diseases/fractures within this book will detail points to address within the history and examination specific to that condition.

HISTORY

PRESENTING COMPLAINT:

This is a one-liner. *Why has the patient presented to hospital?*

e.g. 'left sided facial swelling', 'elective orthognathic surgery'.

HISTORY OF PRESENTING COMPLAINT:

What is the background story behind the presenting complaint?

For an elective procedure, or sudden trauma this may be short and succinct.

The mnemonic SOCRATES is often used to investigate symptoms of pain, but can be applied to other presenting complaints.

- **S** – SITE – where is the pain (mass)?
- **O** – ONSET – did the pain start suddenly, or develop slowly?
- **C** – CHARACTER – describe the pain i.e. is the pain sharp or aching (is the mass firm or soft)? With infections: is there any associated swelling? Or dysphagia/dysphonia?
- **R** – RADIATION – does the pain radiate anywhere?
- **A** – ATTENUATING FACTORS – does anything make the pain better?
- **T** – TIME – when did the pain start? How long has it been present?
- **E** – EXACERBATING FACTORS – does anything make the pain worse?
- **S** – SEVERITY – how bad is the pain? On a scale of 1–10.

In trauma patients it is often worth noting what they perceive to be wrong.

i.e. *'I can't eat'*, *'My teeth don't bite correctly'*, *'My lip feels numb.'*

Listen to the patient and you will know what to examine.

PAST MEDICAL HISTORY:

Is there anything else medically wrong with patient?

Have they had any previous or recent operations?

Think about conditions that would affect or preclude a general anesthetic: heart or lung disease, diabetes, hypertension, endocrine conditions, etc.

Have they had a general anaesthetic before and do they have any potential airway concerns?

Use a 'systems approach', asking questions specific to the following areas:

Cardiovascular, Respiratory, Gastrointestinal, Urogenital, Neurological, Musculoskeletal.

Always document and check tetanus status.

DRUG HISTORY:

- Does the patient have any known drug allergies e.g. Penicillin derivatives? If patient claims to be allergic, ask what happens when they take the medication i.e. severe/mild allergy or an intolerance?
- Ask about current regular medications.

SOCIAL HISTORY:

- Smoking, alcohol use and any recreational drug use
- Marital status, children
- Employment

EXAMINATION

TRAUMA

For emergency admissions the area to be examined may be obvious (i.e. the face) and you may not have time to do a full examination at first. Always remember to document the level of consciousness in all trauma patients using the Glasgow Coma Scale (GCS) (see 'Head Injuries' page 59). For pre-operative elective patients a quick routine full examination is a key skill to learn. While the long lists below for each system appear daunting they will soon become second nature. For the examination sequence specific to site or suspected fracture see the relevant section within this book.

GENERAL INSPECTION

Look at the patient – are they comfortable at rest? Are they in pain, or look unwell? Is there any obvious facial asymmetry/bruising/bleeding/laceration? Document these all carefully (as often in interpersonal violence cases, a police report will be written based on this initial documentation).

CARDIOVASCULAR EXAMINATION

- Feel the pulse – rate? rhythm? If abnormal, get an ECG and discuss with a senior medical colleague if you are unable to interpret it.
- Palpate the apex beat, usually found in the mid-clavicular line 5th intercostal space. If abnormal positioning, discuss with a physician in case of possibility of a cardiomyopathy/ventricular hypertrophy.
- Auscultate the heart in the four areas (Fig 1.1a) and listen for normal heart sounds or any murmurs/abnormal heart sounds. If present, are they occurring in diastole or systole? If having difficulty, ask the patient to hold in a breath and/or lean forward.
- Measure and document the patient's blood pressure.

RESPIRATORY EXAMINATION

- Examine the hands, look for clubbing and nicotine staining
- Inspect the patient; are there any scars on the anterior or posterior chest wall?
- Palpate the chest wall to assess equal and bilateral rib expansion
- Percussion – tap onto a flattened finger placed on the skin. Is the sound hollow or dull?
- Auscultate for breathing sounds. Three sites on each side of the chest, front and back, comparing each side (Fig 1.1a). Listen for normal breathing sounds and added sounds, such as crackles/crepitations (e.g. Pneumonia, Pulmonary Oedema) or a wheeze (e.g. Asthma).

ABDOMINAL EXAMINATION

- Inspect the abdomen for scars or obvious masses.
- Palpate for pain in each of the nine areas of the abdomen (Fig 1.1b). First superficially and then move deep and press harder. Always looking at the patient to check for facial expressions indicating pain. Can you feel any normal/abnormal masses? If so, think of the underlying anatomy.

- Palpate the lower edge of the liver – is it enlarged? Ask the patient to take a deep breath in and out and move the flat edge of your hand up the patients abdomen to feel the free edge.
- You may wish to ballot the kidneys and attempt to examine for splenomegaly
- Auscultate for bowel sounds in a central area of the abdomen

NEUROLOGICAL EXAMINATION

This involves a complex assessment of general neurology and is beyond the scope of this text. For a thorough description of general neurological examination, please consult an appropriate text.

- Cranial nerve examination: Facial nerve function may be of extreme importance in certain pre-operative patients/lacerations and trauma to the face, trigeminal nerve deficit may indicate a fracture with associated nerve injury.
- Assess Tone, Power, Co-ordination, Reflexes and Sensation of all four limbs.

AT THE END OF YOUR HISTORY AND EXAMINATION BE SURE TO:

- Document a diagnosis or impression
- Outline a plan of further action i.e. blood tests, radiographs, IV fluids, etc.
- Record any discussion regarding management you have had with your on-call senior
- Sign, date and time every clinical entry.

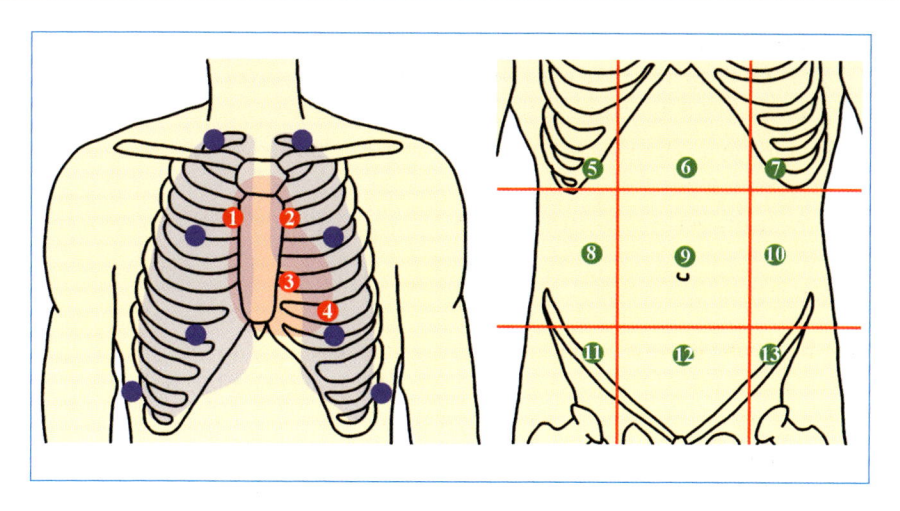

Fig 1.1. a) Cardiac (red dots) and Pulmonary (blue dots) auscultation sites, b) Regions for abdominal palpation (green dots).

1. Aortic valve – 2nd intercostal space, right sternal edge.
2. Pulmonary valve – 2nd intercostal space, left sternal edge.
3. Tricuspid valve – 4th intercostal space, left sternal edge.
4. Mitral valve – 5th intercostal space, mid-clavicular line.
5. Right hypochondriac region
6. Epigastric region
7. Left hypochondriac region
8. Right lumbar region
9. Umbilical region
10. Left lumbar region
11. Right inguinal region
12. Hypogastric region
13. Left inguinal region

AN INTRODUCTION TO TEETH

The adult human typically has 32 teeth, arranged into upper and lower arches of 8 symmetrical pairs. The most posterior teeth (wisdom teeth) are sometimes congenitally absent. Each tooth is composed of a crown, made of enamel and dentine, containing the pulp chamber, and a root containing root canals connected to the pulp chamber. The tooth morphology varies considerably depending on the position in the arch: anterior teeth have a crown and a single root whereas posterior teeth have more complex crowns composed of several cusps and have either single or multiple roots. In general, the crown is visible above the gum (gingiva) and the roots are buried beneath the gingival margin within the alveolar bone. Cementum lines the root surface and attaches to the bone via the periodontal ligament. The terms coronal (close to the crown) and apical (close to the apex of the root) are typically used to describe positions relative to the long axis of the tooth.

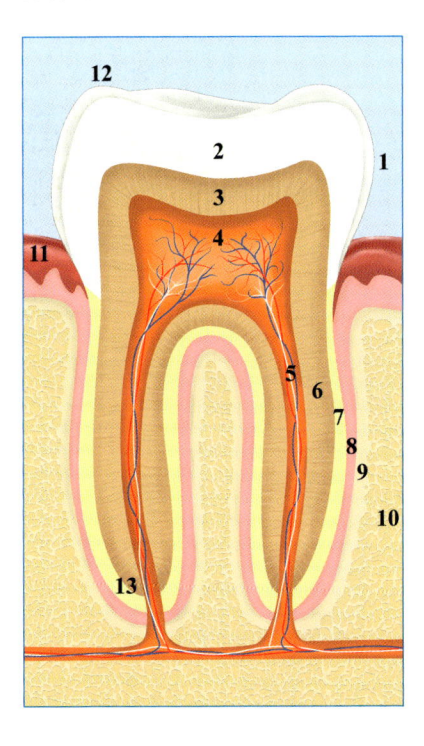

Fig 1.2. Picture of a typical multi-rooted tooth and the tooth-supporting tissues.

1. *Crown*
2. *Enamel*
3. *Dentine*
4. *Pulp cavity containing neurovascular pulp tissue*
5. *Root canal containing neurovascular bundle*
6. *Root*
7. *Cementum*
8. *Periodontal ligament*
9. *Lamina dura of alveolar bone tooth socket*
10. *Cancellous alveolar bone*
11. *Gingiva*
12. *Cusp*
13. *Apex of root*

Whilst an adult typically has 32 teeth, a young child has only 20, with 5 symmetrical pairs arranged in each of the upper and lower arches. These teeth are called deciduous teeth (primary teeth) and are colloquially referred to as 'milk teeth' or 'baby teeth.' These teeth exfoliate (fall out naturally) as the permanent teeth begin to erupt.

NUMBERING TEETH

Dental nomenclature can seem daunting at first, but it does follow straightforward principles. The mouth is divided in 4 quadrants based on their anatomical position in the patient. Each quadrant has 8 teeth, which are numbered 1 to 8 starting at the midline (Fig 1.3).

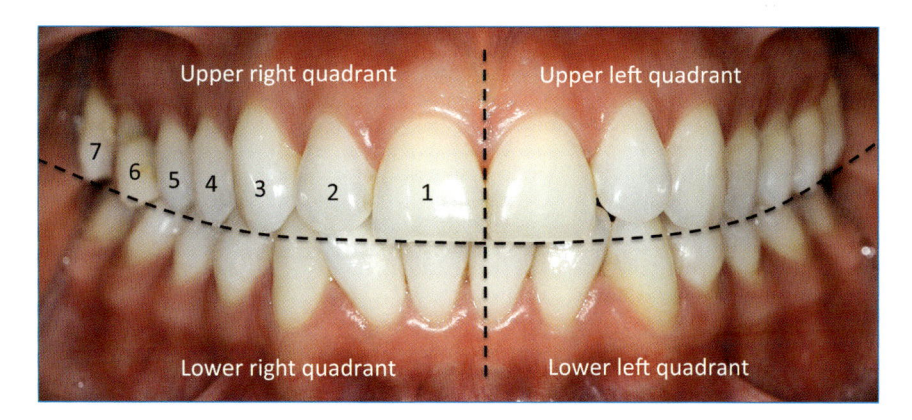

Fig 1.3. Labelling the quadrants of the mouth and numbering the teeth

1. *Central incisor*
2. *Lateral incisor*
3. *Canine*
4. *First premolar*
5. *Second premolar*
6. *First molar*
7. *Second molar*
8. *Third molar/wisdom tooth (missing in this patient)*

The terms mesial and distal are used to describe positions in relation to the midline of the arch. Mesial refers to a position along the arch that is closer to the midline. Distal refers to a position along the arch that is further from the midline. There are 2 commonly used shorthand notation systems used to name teeth. These are the Zsigmondy-Palmer system and the FDI system.

ZSIGMONDY-PALMER SYSTEM

In this system, each quadrant is denoted in relation to a cross as shown:

UPPER RIGHT QUADRANT 8 7 6 5 4 3 2 1	UPPER LEFT QUADRANT 1 2 3 4 5 6 7 8
8 7 6 5 4 3 2 1 LOWER RIGHT QUADRANT	1 2 3 4 5 6 7 8 LOWER LEFT QUADRANT

Individual teeth can also be described in this manner, using only the section of the cross that corresponds to the quadrant within which the tooth in question is located, or abbreviations for the quadrant are used:

$$\underline{5}|$$

Upper right 2nd premolar: UR5

$$\overline{3\,7}|$$

Lower left canine and 2nd molar: LL3 LL7

In children, the Zsigmondy-Palmer method uses the same notation of quadrants but deciduous teeth are lettered A through to E, from the midline distally (there are no premolar teeth or 3rd molar teeth in the deciduous dentition).

A = deciduous central incisor

B = deciduous lateral incisor

C = deciduous canine

D = deciduous first molar

E = deciduous second molar

E D C B A	A B C D E
E D C B A	A B C D E

FDI SYSTEM

The FDI system follows a similar principle as the Zsigmondy-Palmer system, but each quadrant is ascribed a number:

Upper right quadrant 1	Upper left quadrant 2
4 Lower right quadrant	3 Lower left quadrant

When describing the tooth, the number of the appropriate quadrant is recorded followed by the tooth number. For example:

Upper right canine = 1 3

Upper left wisdom tooth = 2 8

Lower left 1st premolar = 3 4

Lower right wisdom tooth = 4 8

In the FDI system, deciduous quadrants are labelled 5-8 and the teeth are given numbers 1–5 from the midline distally:

Upper right quadrant 5	Upper left quadrant 6
8 Lower right quadrant	7 Lower left quadrant

Upper right deciduous canine = 5 3

Upper left deciduous second molar tooth = 6 5

Lower right deciduous canine = 8 3

Lower left deciduous second molar = 7 5

ERUPTION DATES

Tooth eruption is the emergence of the tooth through the gums into the mouth. There is huge variability in eruption dates of both deciduous and permanent teeth and they are notoriously difficult to remember.

In general, teeth erupt symmetrically although the timing of upper and lower teeth eruption varies. Furthermore, as the tooth continues to erupt into its final position, root formation continues, until its completion some 12–24 months after initial eruption of the tooth.

Table 1.1. Deciduous teeth eruption dates

Date of eruption (months after birth)	8	9	18	14	24
Upper deciduous teeth	A	B	C	D	E
Lower deciduous teeth	A	B	C	D	E
Date of eruption (months after birth)	8	7	16	12	20

Table 1.2. Permanent teeth eruption dates

Date of eruption (years after birth)	7	8	11.5	10	11	6	12	18
Upper permanent teeth	1	2	3	4	5	6	7	8
Lower permanent teeth	1	2	3	4	5	6	7	8
Date of eruption (years after birth)	6.5	7	10.5	10	11	6	12	18

A good knowledge of eruption dates, while seemingly laboured, is essential when treating paediatric dental trauma, as the management is different between deciduous and permanent teeth (see 'Dental Trauma' page 72).

DENTAL OCCLUSION

This describes the way teeth meet when a patient bites together. An in-depth discussion of the complex nature of dental occlusion lies outside the scope of this book. However, in the on-call environment, a deranged occlusion, or an abnormal 'bite' may be a sign of an underlying facial injury.

Similarly, a previously deranged occlusion should return to normal after appropriate treatment has been performed, for example it may indicate the successful reduction of a mandibular fracture. As such, it is often essential to assess dental occlusion in the post-operative ward or clinic review.

TERMINOLOGY

- **Overbite** – the vertical overlap of the maxillary and mandibular central incisors. Measured from the tips of the incisors, in mm. Normal overbite is 3–5mm.
- **Overjet** – the horizontal overlap of the maxillary and central incisors. Measured from the tips of the incisors, in mm.
- **Open bite** – when a group of teeth fail to occlude. Can either be anterior or posterior.
- **Crossbite** – when a group of teeth have an altered position compared to the occluding arch i.e. the teeth are buccal or lingual in comparison to the occluding teeth.

In orthognathic surgery, formal classifications of dental occlusion are used to grade facial deformity and outcome of surgery. These are based on the relationship between the upper and lower 1st molar teeth and central incisors, and are briefly described below.

CLASS 1:

This is regarded as normal occlusion. The mesiobuccal cusp of the maxillary first molar is aligned with the buccal groove of the mandibular first molar. The edge of the lower central incisor occludes on or below the middle third of the upper central incisor.

CLASS 2:

Here, the buccal groove of the mandibular first molar is distally positioned to the mesiobuccal cusp of the maxillary first molar. Class 2 malocclusion is subdivided into 2 divisions that relate to the position of the anterior teeth.

Class II, Division 1 is where the maxillary anterior teeth are proclined with a large overjet. Class II, Division 2 is where the maxillary anterior teeth are retroclined with a deep overbite.

CLASS 3:

Here the buccal groove of the mandibular first molar is mesially positioned to the mesiobuccal cusp of the maxillary first molar when the teeth are in occlusion. In this situation, the upper central incisors may rest behind the lower central incisors. This relationship is often referred to as a reverse overjet.

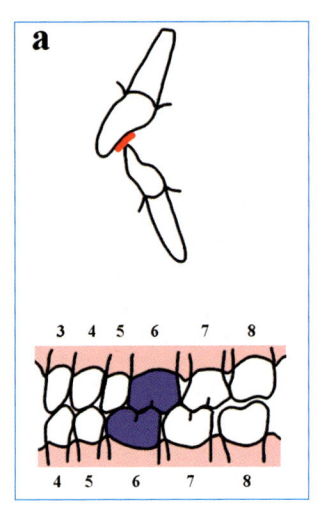

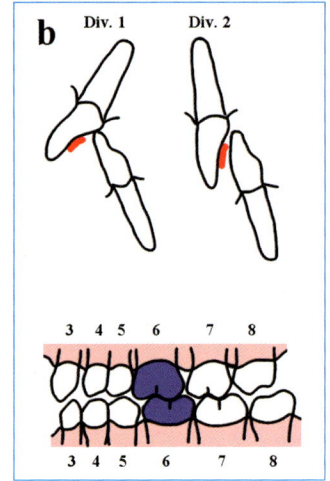

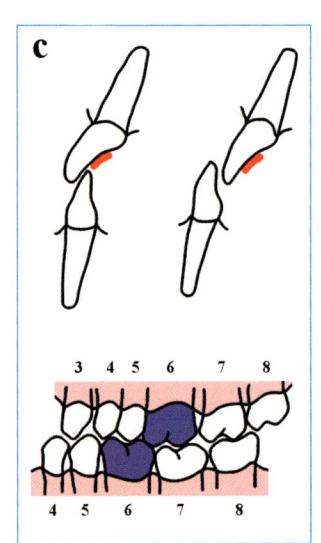

Fig 1.4. Classifications of dental occlusion based upon central incisor and first molar relationships:

   a) *Class I*
   b) *Class II (Division 1 and Division 2)*
   c) *Class III*

ANATOMY

As with all surgical specialties, a good grasp of anatomy is important to provide the basis for sound clinical judgment. In no region of the body is the anatomy more complex than the head and neck and a detailed account of anatomical structures and principles is beyond the scope of this book. However, you should be familiar with the important structures in the head and neck that you will encounter whilst on-call and have exposure to during the procedures you will undertake. Within this sub-section we provide a brief overview of the face and facial skeleton, oral and nasal cavity and the nerves supplying these areas; together with the trauma zones and lymph node levels of the neck.

FACE AND FACIAL SKELETON

As the on-call OMF surgeon, it is vital to be able to accurately describe the face and its important anatomical structures (Fig 1.5). In addition, it is essential to understand the anatomy of the facial skeleton and its relationship to the overlying soft tissue (Fig 1.6). Such knowledge aids with diagnosis of pathology itself and facilitates appropriate clear communication with colleagues and ensures accurate record keeping.

The importance of these soft and hard tissue relationships becomes clear when examining a patient with facial trauma. By eliciting signs and symptoms that may point to an underlying injury, you are able to guide further investigations.

20 ON-CALL IN ORAL AND MAXILLOFACIAL SURGERY

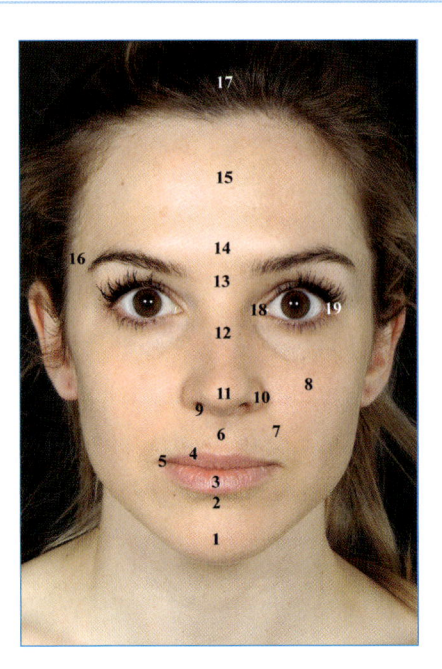

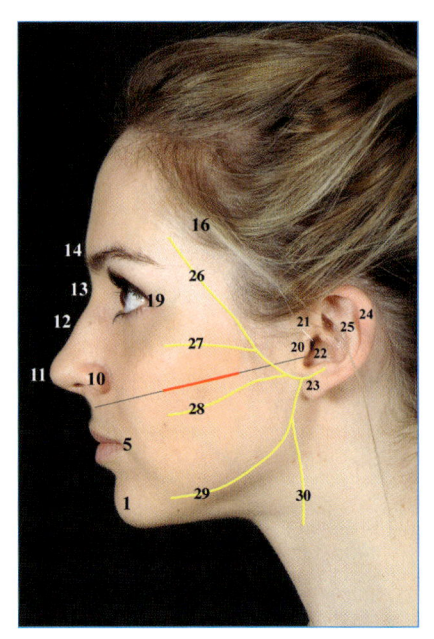

Fig 1.5. (a) Anterior view of surface anatomy of face. (b) Lateral view of surface anatomy of face, with representation of facial nerve (yellow line) and parotid duct (red line – middle third of line drawn from inferior tragus to mid-point of philtrum).

1. Chin
2. Labio-mental groove
3. Vermillion of lower lip
4. Vermillion border of upper lip
5. Oral commissure
6. Philtrum
7. Naso-labial groove
8. Cheek
9. Nares (nostril)
10. Ala of nose
11. Nasal tip
12. Dorsum/bridge of nose
13. Nasion
14. Glabella
15. Forehead
16. Temple
17. Scalp
18. Medial canthus
19. Lateral canthus
20. Tragus
21. External auditory meatus
22. Conchal bowl
23. Lobe
24. Helix
25. Antihelix
26. Temporal branch of facial nerve
27. Zygomatic branch of facial nerve
28. Buccal branch of facial nerve
29. Marginal mandibular branch of facial nerve
30. Cervical branch of facial nerve

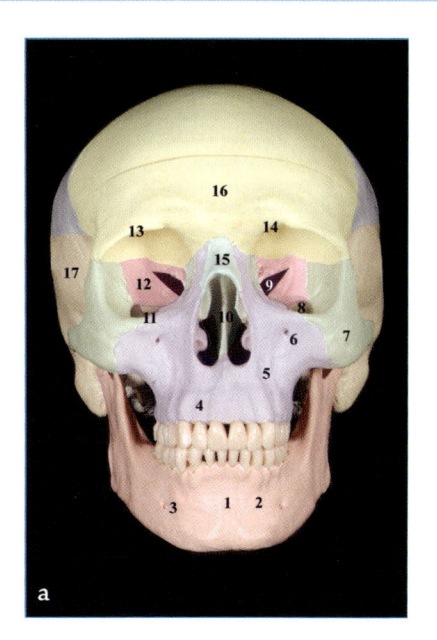

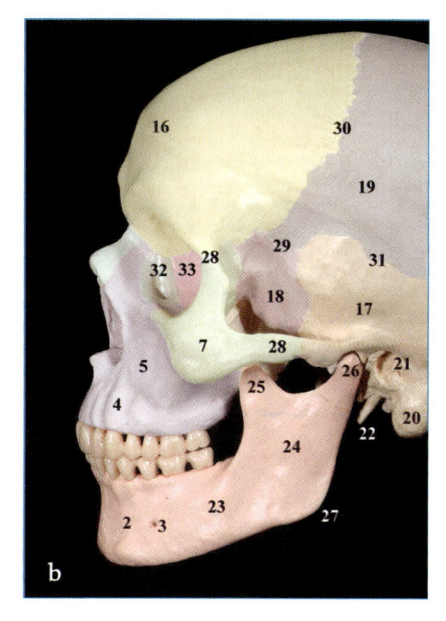

Fig 1.6 (a) Anterior view of skull (b) Lateral view of skull

1. Symphysis of mandible
2. Parasymphysis of mandible
3. Mental foramen
4. Alveolus of maxilla
5. Maxilla
6. Infraorbital foramen
7. Zygoma
8. Infraorbital fissure
9. Supraorbital fissure
10. Septum
11. Infraorbital rim/margin
12. Greater wing of sphenoid (orbital/anterior surface)
13. Supraorbital rim/margin
14. Supraorbital notch
15. Nasal bone
16. Frontal bone
17. Temporal bone
18. Greater wing of sphenoid (temporal/lateral surface)
19. Parietal bone
20. Mastoid process of temporal bone
21. External acoustic meatus
22. Styloid process
23. Body of mandible
24. Ramus of mandible
25. Coronoid process
26. Mandibular condyle
27. Angle of mandible
28. Zygomatico-frontal suture
29. Pterion (union of sphenoid, temporal, frontal and parietal bones)
30. Coronal suture
31. Squamosal suture
32. Lacrimal bone'
33. Ethmoid bone'

ORAL CAVITY, NASAL CAVITY AND PHARYNX

The oral cavity is a complex structure containing both hard and soft tissues. As with the face, you must be able to describe the site of injury and appreciate the anatomy of the nasal cavity and pharynx.

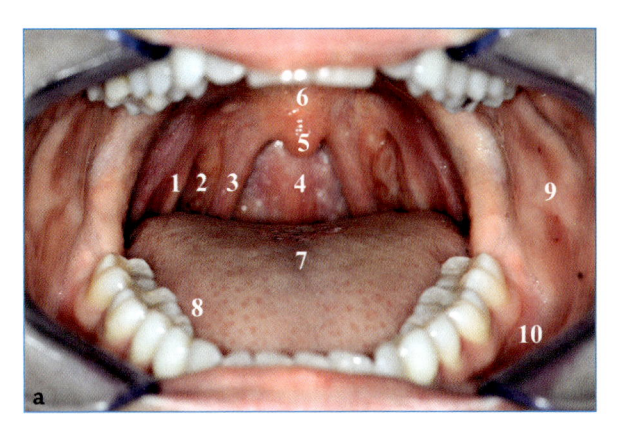

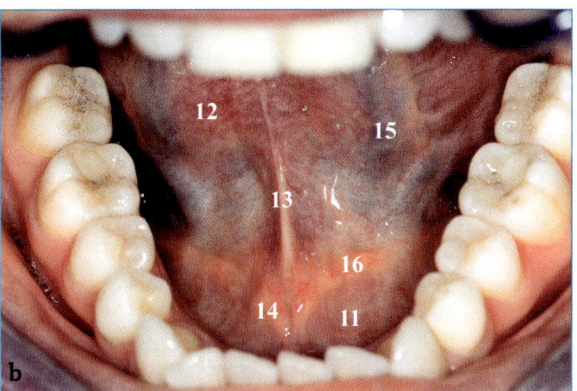

Fig 1.7. a) Intraoral and b) floor of mouth anatomy. The Parotid duct (Stenson's Duct, Fig 1.5b) drains via the Parotid papilla, which is out of sight, opposite the upper second molar teeth bilaterally:

1. Palatoglossal arch
2. Palatine tonsil
3. Palatopharyngeal arch
4. Posterior pharyngeal wall
5. Uvula
6. Soft palate
7. Dorsum of tongue
8. Lateral border of tongue
9. Buccal mucosa
10. Buccal sulcus
11. Floor of mouth
12. Ventral surface of tongue
13. Lingual fraenum
14. Submandibular duct openings
15. Lingual vein
16. Sublingual fold

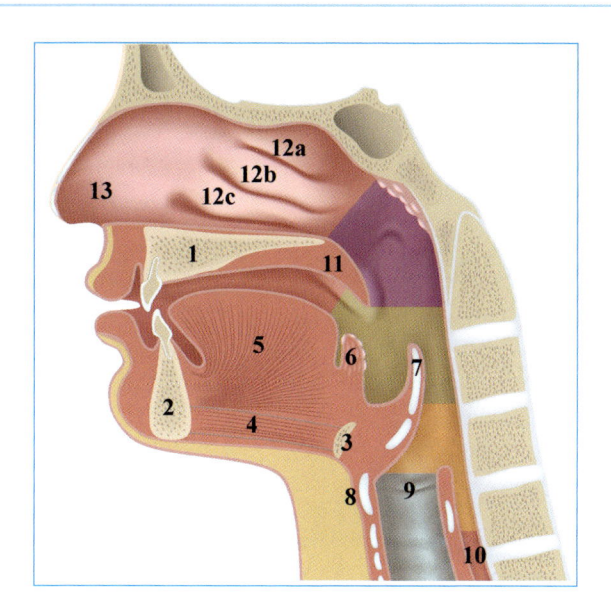

Fig 1.8. Sagittal section to show nasal cavity and pharynx: Nasopharynx (blue), oropharynx (green), laryngopharynx (yellow) and larynx (light blue) shaded.

1. Hard palate
2. Mandible
3. Hyoid bone
4. Geniohyoid muscle
5. Genioglossus muscle
6. Lingual tonsil
7. Epiglottis
8. Thyroid cartilage
9. Vocal fold leading to larynx
10. Oesophagus
11. Soft palate with uvula
12. Superior (a), middle (b) and inferior (c) turbinates (conchae)
13. Little's area/Kiesselbach's plexus (common site of epistaxis)

NERVES OF THE FACE AND ORAL CAVITY

Within OMFS an understanding of the innervation of the facial soft tissue and dentition is essential. The facial nerve (CN VII) innervates the muscles of facial expression, the submandibular and sublingual glands (parasympathetic supply) and provides taste sensation to the anterior two-thirds of the tongue. It has five main branches within the face (Fig 1.5b). The trigeminal nerve (CNV) innervates the muscles of mastication and provides sensation to the face. It has three major divisions (Fig 1.9). As the on-call OMF surgeon this knowledge will be applicable when anaesthetising the face or dentition, for example a nerve block to suture a facial laceration, or tooth anaesthesia in dental trauma (Fig 1.10).

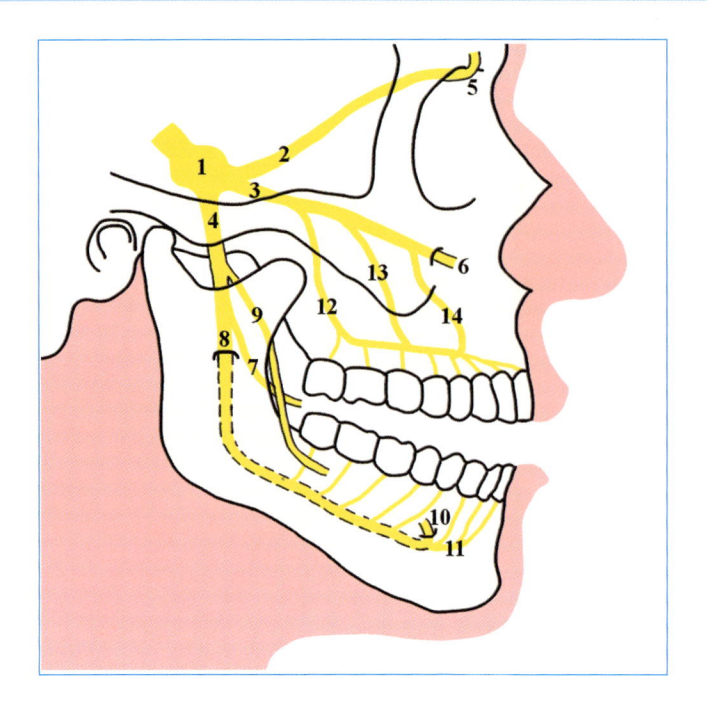

Fig 1.9. Branches of the Trigeminal nerve (CN V).

1. *Trigeminal nerve ganglion*
2. *Ophthalmic nerve (V1)*
3. *Maxillary nerve (V2)*
4. *Mandibular nerve (V3)*
5. *Supraorbital nerve (exiting through supraorbital foramen/notch)*
6. *Infraorbital nerve (exiting through infraorbital foramen)*
7. *Lingual nerve*
8. *Inferior alveolar nerve (entering mandibular canal via mandibular foramen)*
9. *Buccal nerve*
10. *Mental nerve (exiting via mental foramen)*
11. *Incisive nerve*
12. *Posterior superior alveolar nerve*
13. *Middle superior alveolar nerve*
14. *Anterior superior alveolar nerve*

ON-CALL IN ORAL AND MAXILLOFACIAL SURGERY   25

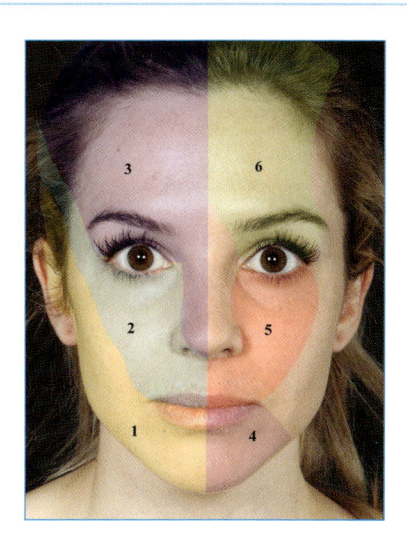

Fig 1.10. Regional innervation of the face (right side) and nerves that can be blocked to achieve facial anaesthesia (left side)

1. Mandibular division of the Trigeminal nerve (V1)
2. Maxillary division of the Trigeminal nerve (V2)
3. Ophthalmic division of the Trigeminal nerve (V3)
4. Mental nerve
5. Infraorbital nerve
6. Supraorbital nerve (and supratrochlear nerve)

ESSENTIALS

THE NECK

The neck has a complex anatomical arrangement. Again, whilst a complete explanation is beyond the scope of this book, its anatomy has some important clinical ramifications. Surface features will act as important landmarks to accurately assess and diagnose traumatic injuries and pathology.

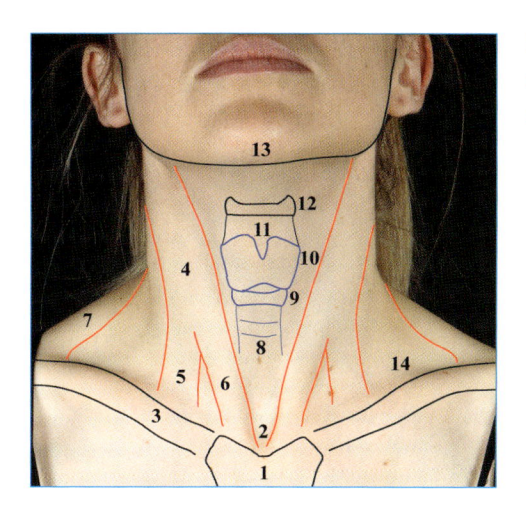

Fig 1.11. Anterior view of neck with superimposed underlying structures

1. Manubrium
2. Jugular notch
3. Clavicle
4. Sternocleidomastoid muscle (SCM)
5. Clavicular head of SCM
6. Sternal head of SCM
7. Trapezius
8. Trachea
9. Cricoid cartilage
10. Thyroid cartilage
11. Thyroid notch
12. Hyoid bone
13. Lower border of mandible
14. Supraclavicular fossa

The neck is anatomically divided into anterior and posterior triangles (Fig 1.12). The anterior triangle of the neck is bounded by the midline of the neck, the lower border of the mandible and the anterior border of SCM. It is subdivided, as shown in Fig 1.12 into the submandibular, submental, carotid and muscular triangle. The posterior triangle of the neck is bounded by the anterior border of sternocleidomastoid, the anterior border of trapezius and the middle third of the clavicle. It is subdivided, as shown in the diagram, into the occipital and supraclavicular triangles. The borders and contents of these triangles are discussed in Table 1.3.

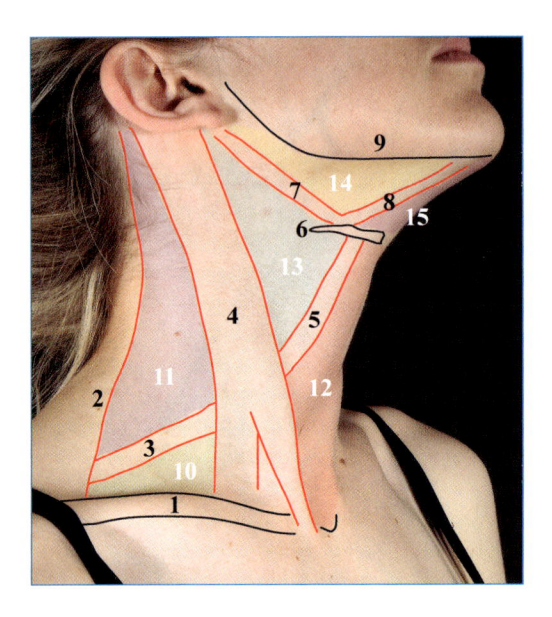

Fig 1.12. Lateral view of neck to display triangles of the neck and the underlying structures comprising their anatomical borders

1. Clavicle
2. Anterior border of Trapezius
3. Inferior belly of Omohyoid
4. SCM
5. Superior belly of Omohyoid
6. Hyoid bone
7. Posterior belly of Digastric
8. Anterior belly of Digastric
9. Lower border of the Mandible
10. Supraclavicular triangle
11. Occipital triangle
12. Muscular triangle
13. Carotid triangle
14. Submandibular triangle
15. Submental triangle

Table 1.3. Triangles of the neck: Anatomical boundaries and contents

Name	Borders	Contents
Anterior triangle		
Submandibular (Fig 1.12 no. 14)	• Superiorly by the lower border of the mandible • Other 2 edges are made of the anterior and posterior bellies of digastric • Floor is the mylohyoid, hypoglossus muscle and middle constrictor muscle	• Submandibular gland • Nerve to mylohyoid • Hypoglossal nerve • Facial artery and vein
Submental (Fig 1.12 no. 15)	• Apex at the mandibular symphysis • Base at the hyoid • Laterally by the left and right anterior bellies of digastric • Floor is the 2 mylohyoid muscles meeting in the middle to form a fibrous raphe • NOTE: this is the only anterior triangle to cross the midline	• Submental lymph nodes • Small blood vessels that form the anterior jugular vein
Carotid (Fig 1.12 no. 13)	• Posteriorly by the anterior aspect of the sternocleidomastoid • Anteriorly by the superior belly of omohyoid • Superiorly by the posterior belly of digastric	• Carotid sheath containing common carotid artery, internal jugular vein and vagus nerve. • Hypoglossal nerve • Superior root of ansa cervicalis • Accessory nerve • Deep cervical lymph nodes • Part of cervical plexus
Muscular (Fig 1.12 no. 12)	• Anteriorly by the midline of the neck • Supero-posteriorly by the superior belly of omohyoid • Inferio-posteriorly by the sternocleidomastoid	• Sternothyroid and sternohyoid muscles • Thyroid gland • Parathyroid glands

ESSENTIALS

Posterior triangle		
Occipital (Fig 1.12 no. 11)	• Anterior aspect of trapezius • Posterior edge of sternocleidomastoid • Inferior belly of omohyoid	• External jugular vein • Posterior branches of cervical plexus • Accessory nerve • Trunks of brachial plexus • Cervical lymph nodes
Supraclavicular (Fig 1.12 no. 10)	• Inferiorly by the clavicle • Superiorly by the inferior belly of omohyoid • Anteriorly by the sternocleidomastoid	• 3rd part of subclavian artery • Supraclavicular artery • Supraclavicular lymph nodes

Two further classifications are important in terms of the clinical problems that are typically encountered by the on-call OMFS team. These include a zonal classification of the neck for the purposes of trauma assessment and the division of the neck into levels based on lymph node drainage.

TRAUMA ZONES OF THE NECK

Penetrating neck injuries have the potential to be life-threatening. A deep injury is indicated when the wound extends deep to platysma. The neck can be divided into 3 trauma zones (Fig 1.13).

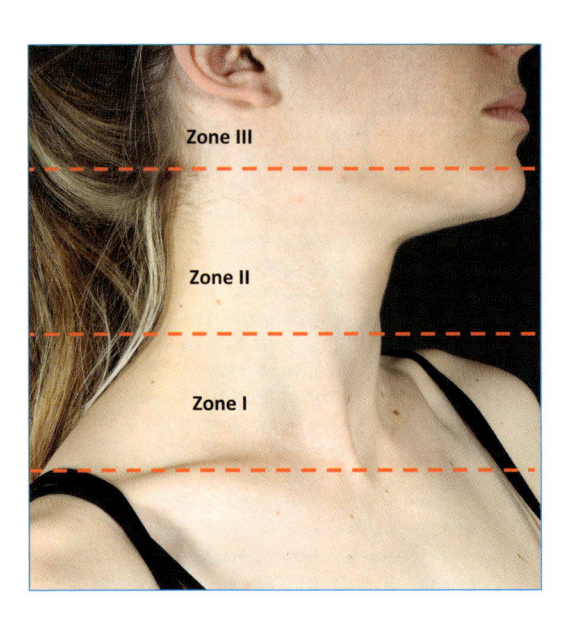

Fig 1.13. Lateral view of neck with markings for trauma zones I-III

Table 1.4. Trauma zones of the neck: Anatomical boundaries and contents

Name	Site	Contents	Notes
Zone 1	Between the horizontal plane passing through cricoid cartilage to level of sternal notch and clavicles	• Proximal common carotid artery • Vertebral artery • Subclavian artery • Subclavian and jugular veins • Trachea • Recurrent laryngeal and vagus nerve • Oesophagus • Thoracic duct	• High mortality due to the proximity to great vessels. • Sternotomy or thoracotomy often required to control haemorrhage
Zone 2	Horizontal plane through angles of mandible down to plane passing through cricoid cartilage	• Carotid arteries • Jugular vein • Pharynx • Larynx • Recurrent laryngeal and vagus nerve • Spinal cord	• Access obtained by simple neck incisions
Zone 3	Between skull base and plane through angles of mandible	• Extracranial carotid and vertebral arteries • Jugular vein • Spinal cord • Glossopharyngeal, Vagus, Accessory and Hypoglossal nerves • Sympathetic truck	• Presence of craniofacial skeleton makes access hard - often requires craniotomy and or mandibulotomy to displace mandible for access. High mortality from vascular injury.

LYMPH NODE LEVELS

Cervical lymphadenopathy is an important diagnostic sign for infection, inflammation or malignancy. Different regions of the head, neck and face drain to different nodal sites. Therefore it is important to be able to describe the level of the affected (enlarged) lymph node (Fig 1.14). Nodal level classification is summarised in table 1.5.

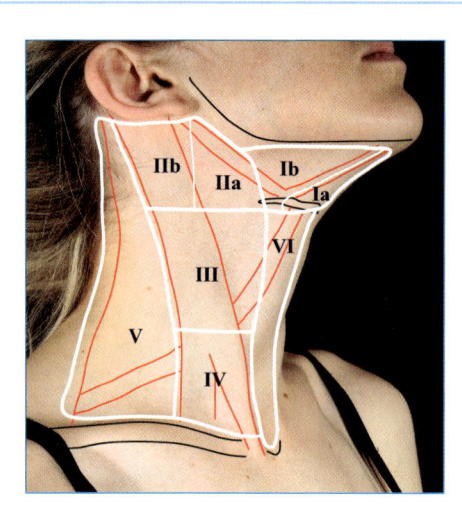

Fig 1.14. Lymph node levels of the neck, with basic representation of underlying anatomy

Table 1.5. Lymph node levels of the neck: Anatomical boundaries and contents

Level	Name	Site	Source of drainage
IA	Submental Group	• Submental triangle	• Floor of mouth • Anterior tongue • Anterior mandibular ridge • Lower lip
IB	Submandibular Group	• Submandibular triangle	• Oral cavity • Anterior nasal cavity • Soft tissues of midface • Submandibular gland
IIA/IIB	Upper Jugular Group	• IIA and IIB are divided vertically by the spinal accessory nerve. • Around upper third of internal jugular between skull base to inferior border of hyoid - anterior to spinal accessory nerve • Medial boundary is lateral border of sternohyoid and posterior boundary is posterior border of SCM.	• Oral and nasal cavities • Nasopharynx • Oropharynx • Hypopharynx • Larynx • Parotid

Level	Name	Site	Source of drainage
III	Middle Jugular Group	• Around the middle third of internal jugular vein • Inferior border of hyoid bone to inferior border of cricoid cartilage. Anteriorly by the sternohyoid and posteriorly by the posterior border of SCM	• Oral cavity • Nasopharynx • Oropharynx • Hypopharynx • Pharynx
IV	Lower Jugular Group	• Lower third of jugular vein from inferior border of cricoid cartilage to clavicle. Anteriorly by the sternohyoid and posteriorly by the SCM	• Hypopharynx • Cervical oesophagus • Larynx
V	Posterior triangle group	• Posterior triangle	• Nasopharynx • Oropharynx • Thyroid gland
VI	Anterior compartment group	• Hyoid bone to suprasternal notch. Lateral boundaries are common carotid arteries. Contains pre- and paratracheal, perithyroidal nodes and nodes around recurrent laryngeal nerve	• Thyroid gland • Larynx • Cervical oesophagus • Apex of piriform sinus.

ESSENTIALS

RADIOLOGY

Radiological investigations should be used to further investigate and support clinical findings rather than to 'fish' for anomalies. Commonly available investigations in the on-call setting are detailed in table 1.6.

Table 1.6. Radiograph views and their clinical indications

Radiographic/Imaging view	What is it useful for?	Notes
Occipitomental (OM) radiograph at 10 and 30 degrees.	Maxilla and maxillary sinus (e.g. fluid level) Orbital margins Zygomatic arch Nasofrontal buttress	
Submentovertex radiograph	Maxilla Supraorbital margin Zygomatic arch	This is rarely used now because of the increased radiation dose required.
Lateral facial radiograph or Lateral cephalogram	Maxilla Pterygoid plates Orthognathic Surgery planning	Highlights dish-face deformity of Le Fort fractures Demonstrates the relationship between the teeth and jaws
Orthopantomogram (OPG)/Dental pantomography (DPT)	Mandible Teeth (periapical infection) Salivary calculi located in submandibular gland	Poor visualization of anterior teeth due to superimposition of c-spine. Requires patient to stand upright and is not always available out of hours (substitute with PA and lateral oblique mandible and obtain OPG in working hours if necessary).
Occlusal radiograph (upper/lower standard occlusals)	Alveolus of anterior teeth. Lower occlusal radiographs can be used to image salivary calculi in the floor-of-mouth.	Evades superimposition artifact seen on OPG.

Radiographic/ Imaging view	What is it useful for?	Notes
Posteroanterior (PA) mandible radiograph	Mandible and specifically, condylar fractures.	Horizontal displacement of mandibular fragments and condylar fragments.
Lateral oblique radiograph	Body, angle, condyle of mandible	Patients who cannot stand for an OPG. Similarly can be used in young children
Computed Tomography (CT)	Facial skeleton (complex facial fractures) Soft tissue collections	Detailed delineation of fragments (and identification of vascular injury with/without contrast enhancement – discuss with radiologist if significant vascular injury suspected). Particularly useful for imaging the orbit and its contents as well as the naso-ethmoidal complex, and in suspected complex midface fractures. It also identifies the location of soft tissue collections and associated airway changes
Magnetic Resonance Imaging (MRI)	Soft tissue structures TMJ	Provides high resolution imaging of complex soft issue structures including vessels, nerves, nodes and thyroid gland. Can't be used in many patients with metallic implants.
Ultrasound scan (USS)	Soft tissue fluid collections, neck space swellings.	Particularly when clinical and other radiological findings are not clear as to whether there is a soft tissue fluid collection which can be drained. Similarly, some collections can be drained through ultrasound-guided needle aspiration by the radiologist.

ESSENTIALS

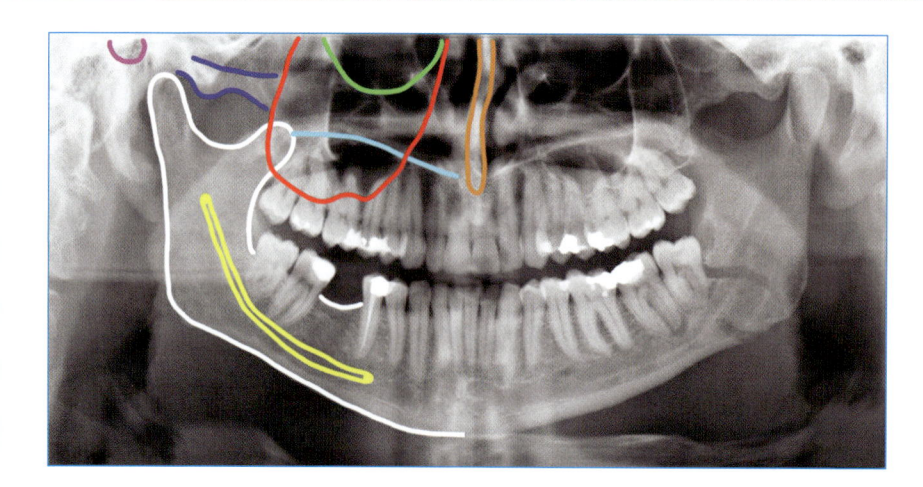

Fig 1.15. An OPG with right sided structures outlined in colour. Note the several restorations (fillings) in the upper and lower teeth, with a root canal treatment in LR5 and a left sided angle of mandible fracture:

- White line – Outline of mandible
- Yellow line – Mandibular canal (containing ID nerve) with mandibular foramen (superior) and mental foramen (inferior) circled
- Red line – Maxillary antrum
- Light blue line – Hard palate
- Dark blue line – Zygomatic arch
- Orange line – Nasal septum
- Green line – Inferior orbital rim
- Purple line – External acoustic meatus

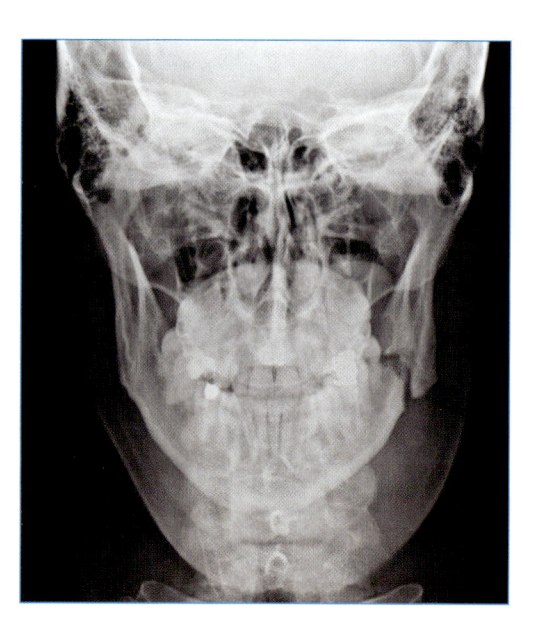

Fig 1.16. A PA mandible taken of the same patient as in the OPG in Fig 1.15. Note the left angle of mandible fracture and the displacement of the two fracture ends not visible on the OPG.

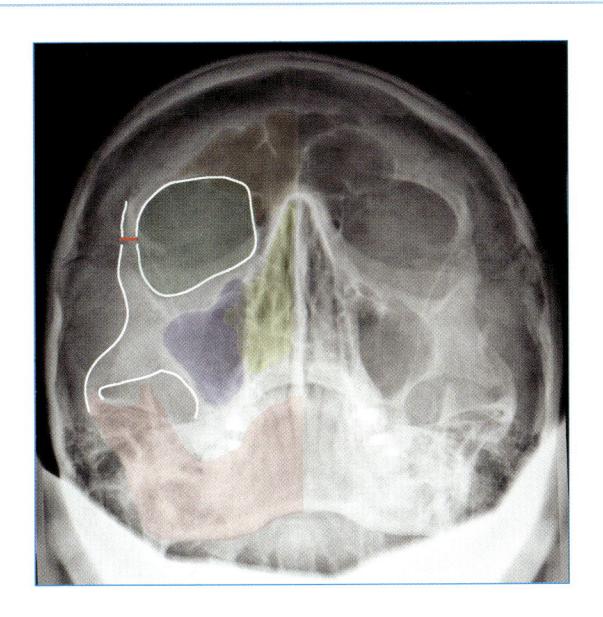

Fig 1.17. OM 10° with anatomy highlighted on right side:

- Red – Mandible
- Blue – Maxillary antrum
- Yellow – Nasal and ethmoid air spaces
- Green – Orbit
- Orange – Frontal Sinus
- White line – Zygomatic arch and orbital rim
- Red line – Zygomatico-frontal suture

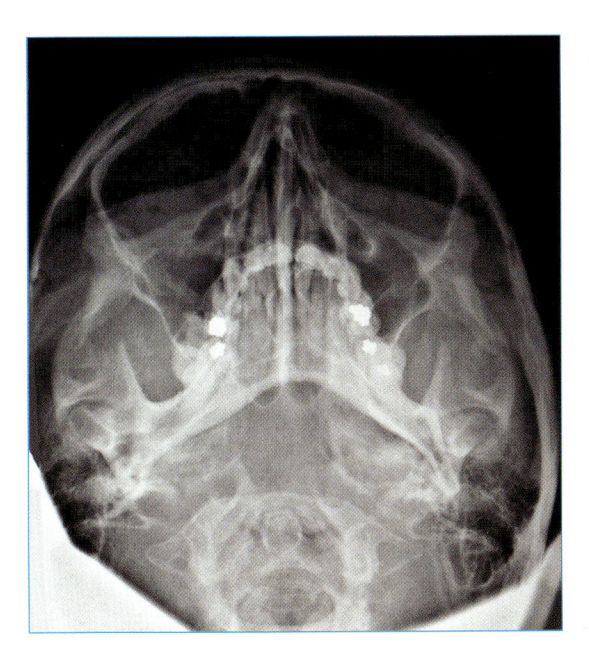

Fig 1.18. OM 30°

36 ON-CALL IN ORAL AND MAXILLOFACIAL SURGERY

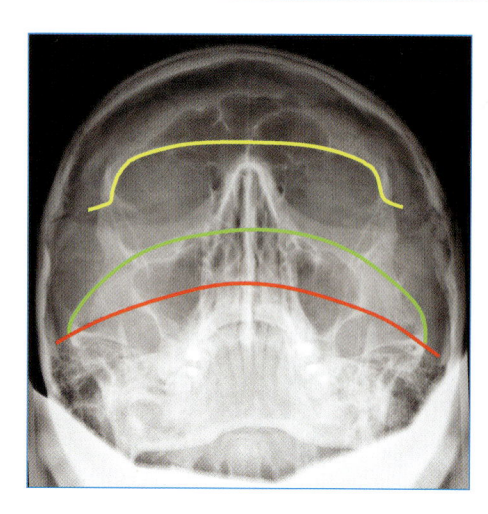

ESSENTIALS

Fig 1.19. OM 10° with McGriggor-Campbell fracture lines superimposed. These lines are to be traced by the radiograph interpreter to aid fracture diagnosis:

- Yellow (Upper) line – passes through the zygomatico-frontal sutures and passes through the supraorbital rims.
- Green (Middle) line – Follows the zygomatic arch and passes through the infraorbital rims.
- Red (Lower) line – Passes through the Mandibular condyle and coronoid process and then though the lateral and medial walls of the maxillary antrum

Fig 1.20. An example of the use of CT to aid facial fracture diagnosis, especially in complex/comminuted fractures. (a)(b) Transverse plane CT with a classic 'tripod' zygomatic complex fracture evident. Also note the left sided peri-orbital soft tissue swelling and surgical emphysema in (a).

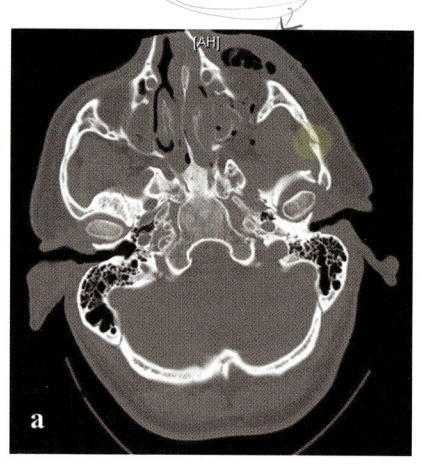

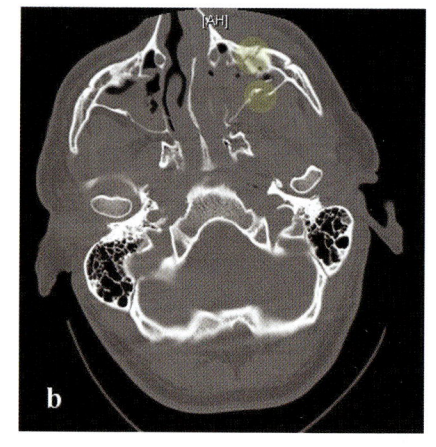

DRUGS

ANALGESICS

When prescribing analgesics for pain you should adhere to the World Health Organisation 'pain ladder'. This describes a stepwise approach, starting at weaker analgesics moving through the different strength opioids.

1. Non-opioid

Paracetamol 1g PO/IV qds +/- NSAID

Ibuprofen 400mg PO tds, MAX 2.4g daily

Aspirin 300-900mg PO 4-6 hrly, MAX 4g daily

N.B. use NSAIDs with extreme caution in patients with renal or hepatic impairment, a history of cardiovascular disease and head injuries. Consult the medical team if in doubt.

2. Weak Opioid

Codeine Phosphate 30-60mg PO/IM 4 hrly, MAX 240mg daily

Dihydrocodeine 30mg PO 4-6 hrly

Tramadol 50-100mg PO/IM/IV 4hrly, MAX 400mg daily

3. Strong Opioid

Morphine sulphate oral liquid (Oramorph) 5-10mg 4hrly, max 1hrly

Morphine SC/IV 5-10mg 4 hourly, max 1hrly (with an antiemetic such as Cyclizine 50mg IV tds or Ondansetron 4-8mg IV tds).

Oxynorm (oral Oxycodone) 5mg PO 4-6hrly, titrate as necessary MAX 400mg daily

Oxycodone 1-10mg IV 4hrly

When using Morphine to manage acute pain it is acceptable to titrate up the dose by 5-10mg every 30 minutes to achieve adequate pain control. Be aware of the risk of opiate overdose, its symptoms and acute management. Use an initial dose of 2.5-5mg in frail or elderly patients. Your hospital will likely have approved pain guidelines to refer to; as such the above should be used as guidance only. N.B. use opiates with caution in patients with/suspected head injury.

ANTIBIOTICS

The antibiotics listed below are not an exhaustive list, but should be the main agents you will encounter. Your hospital should have approved antibiotic guidelines detailing specific dose regimens for each infection.

Amoxicillin	- PO 250 -500mg bd (depending on severity of infection). - IM/IV 500mg tds. IV 1g qds in severe infection
Benzylpenicillin	- IV 0.6-1.2g qds (depending on severity of infection)
Co-amoxiclav	- PO 625mg tds. - IV 1.2g tds (Amoxicillin + Clavulinic Acid, Augmentin™)
Cefuroxime	- PO 250-500mg bd (depending on severity of infection) - IM/IV 750mg -1.5g tds (depending on severity of infection)
Metronidazole	- PO 200-500mg tds - IV 500mg tds
Flucloxacillin	- PO/IM 250-500mg qds - IV 0.25-2g qds
Clindamycin	- PO 150 -450mg qds (depending on severity of infection) - IV 0.6-2.7g daily in 2-3 divided doses - MAX 4.8g in life-threatening infection
Clarithromycin Erythromycin	- PO 250 -500mg qds MAX 4g daily in divided doses in severe infection - IV 12.5mg/kg qds in severe infection

ANTIEMETICS

Post-operative nausea and vomiting is common. Prescribing an antiemetic, as per required, for all patients is recommended. It is important to note that each antiemetic has a specific mode of action, as detailed in the table below. Therefore escalating one drug to a similar mode of action drug is unlikely to alleviate the symptoms of the patient.

Cyclizine	PO/IM/IV 50mg tds	antihistamine
Prochlorperazine	PO 20mg initially, then 10mg 2hrly. IM 12.5mg qds	antidopaminergic
Buccastem®	(buccal prochlorperazine) 3mg tds	antidopaminergic
Ondansetron	PO/IM/IV 4mg tds	$5HT_3$ receptor antagonist
Domperidone	PO 10-20mg tds	antidopaminergic/ prokinetic
Metoclopramide	PO/IM/IV 10mg tds	prokinetic

ORAL SURGERY INSTRUMENTS

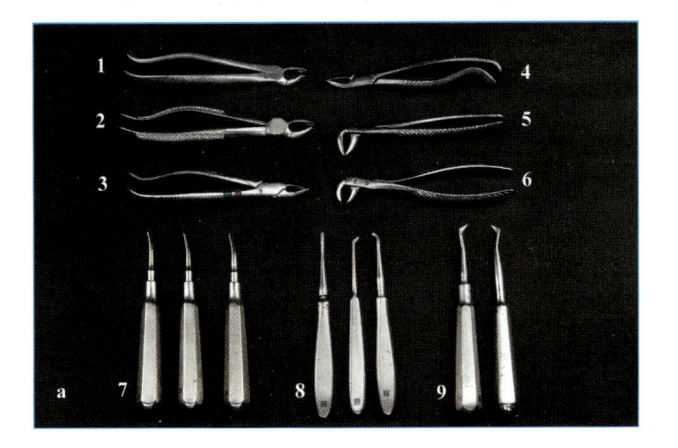

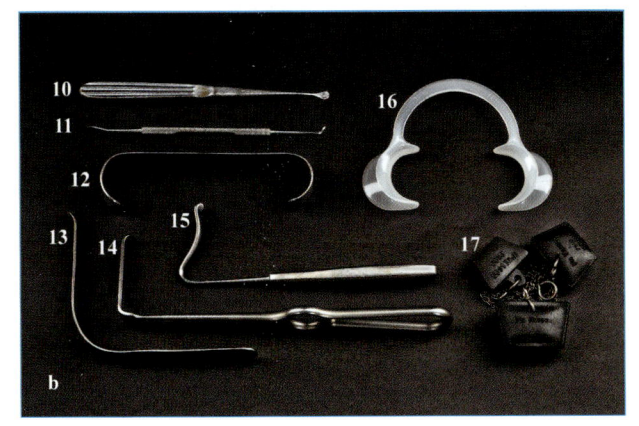

Fig 1.21. (a) and (b) Oral surgery instruments:

1. Upper right molar forceps
2. Upper left molar forceps
3. Upper premolar forceps
4. Upper root forceps
5. Lower root forceps
6. Lower molar forceps
7. Couplands elevators. From left to right - numbers 1,2 and 3
8. Warwick James elevators. From left to right - straight, left and right
9. Cryers elevators. Left and right
10. Wards periosteal elevator
11. Mitchells trimmer
12. Kilner cheek retractor
13. Laster retractor
14. Langenbeck retractor
15. Rake retractor
16. Panoramic mouth prop
17. Mouth props/bite blocks

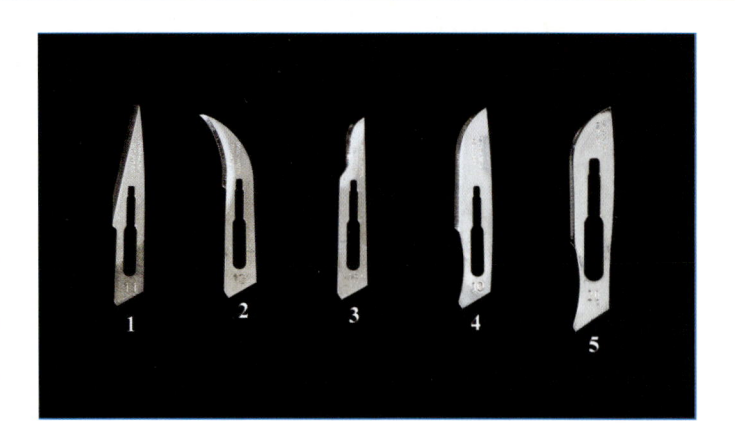

Fig 1.22. Surgical blades:
1. 11 blade
2. 12 blade
3. 15 blade
4. 10 blade
5. 20 blade

EMERGENCY DEPARTMENT

ASSESSMENT AND INITIAL MANAGEMENT OF FACIAL TRAUMA

This section will discuss the general assessment of a patient presenting with facial trauma and its initial management. Specific hard and soft tissue injuries are discussed in turn elsewhere in this chapter.

HISTORY

In addition to a full medical history (see 'Admission Clerking' page 7), important questions include:

- Mechanism of injury? i.e. punch, kick, object, etc.
- Time of injury?
- Any other injuries?
- Any evidence of intracranial injury (Loss of consciousness (LOC) at scene, duration of LOC, nausea/vomiting/headache)?
- Any diplopia/other visual disturbance (suggesting orbital or intracranial injury)?
- Any facial numbness/weakness (nerve deficit)?
- Any rough (fractured) teeth?
- Any malocclusion (maxillary/mandibular fracture)?
- Any previous maxillofacial injury (explaining deformity/radiographic findings etc.)?

EXAMINATION

To examine the face you should follow the routine of inspection and palpation of all areas of the face in a thorough systematic fashion as shown below, so as not to miss subtle findings. Positive findings can be supported by relevant investigations once you have identified possible pathology.

GENERAL INSPECTION

- Wounds, bleeding, contamination
- Burns
- Swelling, ecchymoses
- Facial asymmetry

CRANIUM AND EARS
- Palpate for deformity or depressions
- Inspect the external auditory canal for otorrhoea* and consider otoscopy (a haemotympanum may be suggestive of a basal skull fracture or condylar fracture)
- Assess the ears for soft tissue injury, in particular lacerations and pinna haematomas (see 'Pinna haematoma' page 186)

FRONTAL
- Palpate for deformity
- Assess supraorbital numbness to light touch (CN V1 paraesthesia)

ORBIT

This forms part of the examination of frontal, nasal, zygomatic and maxillary bones. An eye that is swollen shut needs to be examined in order to ensure you do not miss a retrobulbar haemorrhage/orbital compartment syndrome or orbital floor fracture in children, or those patients who have a history of direct ocular injury.

- Looking from above the patient inspect the globes for proptosis (which may suggest retrobulbar haemorrhage)
- Is there any subconjunctival haemorrhage (frequently present with orbital floor fractures)
- Inspect for epiphora (overflow of tears onto the face, which may suggest possible damage to nasolacrimal drainage system)
- Assess eye movements by asking the patient to follow your index finger, moved in an 'H' shape through the centre and extremes of vertical and horizontal gaze. Ensure that the patient keeps his or her head still. Whilst checking this, ask about diplopia (if abnormal may suggest extraocular muscle entrapment or raised ICP). *NB: diplopia can be normal in some individuals in the very extremes of vertical/lateral gaze. If in doubt, discuss with the ophthalmologist or the on-call senior.*
- Palpate the peri-orbital tissues and eyelids for surgical emphysema
- Palpate entire orbital rim for tenderness, bony steps or crepitus (this may suggest a fracture)
- Assess pupillary reaction to light and accommodation (if abnormal it may suggest a raised ICP or isolated CNII or III deficit). To assess the light reflex, place the edge of your non-dominant hand along the bridge of the nose. Assess the direct pupillary response (constriction with

the pen-torch shining at the pupil) and indirect pupillary response (constriction of the contralateral pupil when shining on the ipsilateral pupil). This should be performed in both eyes. Pupillary response to accommodation can be observed with constriction as you move your finger (visual target) away from the patient.
- Consider fundoscopy to assess for retinal haemorrhages or papilloedema
- Assess visual acuity using a Snellen chart. With a standard Snellen chart, this involves covering the non-tested eye with the patient's hand and assessing which numbered line is readable by the patient at a distance of 6 metres from the chart. This should be performed in both eyes so a comparison can be made between the affected and unaffected orbit. The number against the lowest line readable should be documented against the distance read from the chart. For example, normal visual acuity would allow the patient to read the line labelled '6' at 6 metres and should be recorded as '6/6'. The acuity for a patient who can read the line labelled 24 at 6 metres should be recorder as '6/24.' Some Snellen charts use Imperial units (20 feet instead of 6 metres), in which case the same line would be recorded as '20/20'. *Modified and hand-held versions of the Snellen chart can be used but ensure to document the acuity as per the manufacturer's advice.*

NASAL

- Inspect for deviation of nasal bones and/or septum
- Inspect for flattening of nasal bridge and increased inter-canthal distance (i.e. medial canthal ligament disruption in NOE complex fracture)
- Inspect for rhinorrhoea* (basal skull fracture) and epistaxis
- Palpate for bony tenderness and crepitus
- Assess the patency of each nostril (ask the patient if any change from previously)
- Using a nasal speculum inspect for clots or a septal haematoma (see 'Septal haematoma' page 188)

ZYGOMA

- Inspect for flattening of the malar prominence
- Check for trismus due to impaction of coronoid process under fractured arch on opening mandible and in lateral excursion
- Palpate for bony tenderness and crepitus

MAXILLA

Extraoral

- Inspect for deformity (dish-face appearance with Le Fort type fractures) and facial asymmetry (CN VII deficit) or facial lacerations
- Palpate for bony tenderness and crepitus
- Assess for infraorbital nerve numbness (CN V2 deficit)

Intraoral

- Inspect for malocclusion of maxillary origin
- Inspect for missing or fractured teeth
- Palpate for defects, tenderness or crepitus of the hard palate
- Attempt gentle anteroposterior, vertical and lateral distraction of the maxilla by carefully grasping the maxilla (with the thumb placed above the upper central incisors and index finger inside the palate) and attempting to move the upper jaw. Ideally **do this only once** and document any movement to avoid causing bleeding at the fracture site. If any movement, palpate the face for steps or mobile fracture components to localize extent of fracture (i.e. low fracture with 'floating palate', pyramidal type or craniofacial dysjunction).

MANDIBLE

Extraoral

- Assess mouth opening (record MIO in mm)
- Inspect for lower facial swelling or deformity
- Palpate for a step deformity at the lower border of the mandible and bony tenderness
- Palpate over the TMJ
- Apply pressure to the chin with the mouth open (pain may indicate underlying fracture)
- Assess for numbness of the lower lip (suggesting an inferior alveolar nerve (CN V3) deficit).

Intraoral

- Inspect for a sublingual haematoma (this is a fractured mandible until proven otherwise)
- Inspect for dental trauma or a step deformity in the teeth
- Palpate for a step deformity in the mandible
- Assess the patient's occlusion. Premature contact of molar teeth, lateral excursion or an anterior open bite may indicate bilateral

displaced condylar fractures. Some patients may have pre-existing malocclusions so it is important to check this with them.

NECK EXAMINATION
- Inspect the neck for any wounds, swellings or other changes. Note the location of your findings according to the triangle/trauma zone of the neck (as appropriate) (see Fig 1.12/1.13 pages 26 and 28).

TOP TIPS
*Note: At the bedside, differentiate CSF from nasal/aural secretions:
1. Dipstick for glucose (CSF should be positive for glucose, nasal fluid should not)
2. Bloodstained CSF does not clot, blood should (unless on anticoagulants/antiplatelets!)
3. The mixing of blood and CSF also gives a characteristic 'tramline' appearance
4. CSF onto filter paper gives concentric rings, blood does not (not a very sensitive test!)

Additionally, send a sample to the lab to test for Beta 2 Transferrin (>94% sensitive and >98% specific for CSF).

INITIAL MANAGEMENT
At presentation, the patient should be managed according to ATLS® protocol so that life-threatening injuries/complications are prioritised. In a patient with facial injuries, pay particular attention to any airway compromise and/or haemorrhage:

SECURING THE AIRWAY
If there is any doubt in the security of the airway seek help from the on-call anaesthetist immediately. In such circumstances the patient may require a 'definitive airway' (a tube inserted into the trachea beyond the airway-compromising pathology, with an inflated cuff). On the rare occasion that endotracheal intubation is unsuccessful a surgical cricothyroidotomy may be required, with/without a temporary needle cricothyroidotomy in the interim.

One of the common insults to the airway in facial fractures is uncontrolled haemorrhage. The following methods are available to control bleeding:

CONTROLLING HAEMORRHAGE

- **Bilateral mouth props/bite blocks.** These are used in an emergency to tamponade midfacial bleeding and protect the airway (Fig 2.1).
- **Nasal packing.** If there is epistaxis threatening the airway, you may be asked to pack the nose before your seniors arrive (see 'Nasal packing' page 180).
- **Bridle Wiring.** If the patient has a bleeding mandibular fracture which is complicating the airway, or a mobile mandible fracture (e.g. bilateral parasymphysis fractures) allowing the tongue to fall back posteriorly, consider performing a bridle wire procedure to tamponade the fracture and maintain the airway (see 'Bridle wring' page 178).

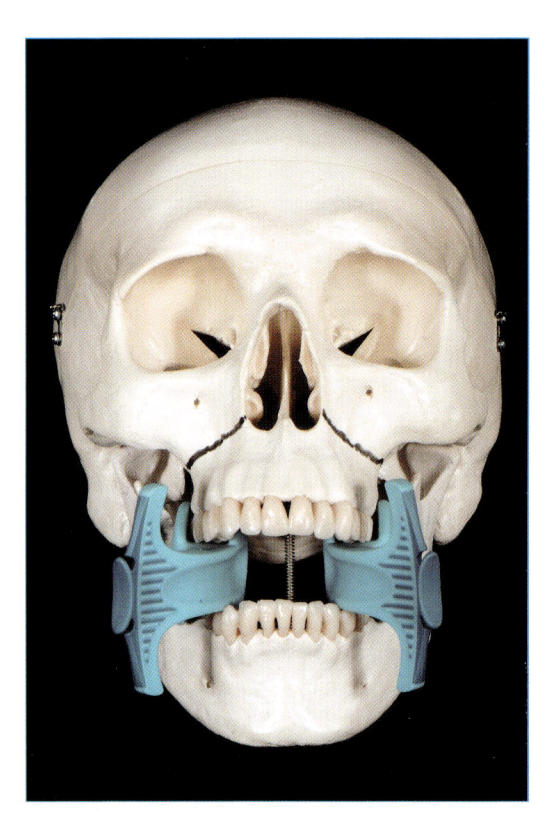

Fig 2.1. Representation of bilateral mouth props/bite blocks, placed to tamponade the bleeding from a Le Fort I midfacial fracture

FURTHER MANAGEMENT

Once the assessment and initial management is complete, findings from the history and examination may prompt investigations to aid diagnosis:

- Blood tests – Full Blood Count, Urea and Electrolytes (Biochemistry), Coagulation Screen, Group and Screen (+/- other tests relevant to the history and examination).
- Radiographic investigations (see 'Radiology' page 32).
- If the patient is to be admitted, then it is appropriate to discuss the patient with your senior to either check that your management is appropriate or arrange for them to review the patient if needed.

MIDFACIAL FRACTURES

ANATOMY AND CLASSIFICATION

The middle third of the facial skeleton is composed of a group of bones forming a three-dimensional structure of vertical and transverse functional buttresses. Therefore when managing midfacial fractures, restoration of the integrity of these buttresses is required to ensure a successful outcome.

The vertical buttresses are key in resisting vertical/masticatory forces and are named as follows: (Fig 2.2)

1. Nasofrontal (alveolar process of maxilla to frontal bone)
2. Zygomatic (zygoma to frontal bone)
3. Pterygomaxillary (sitting posteriorly, maxillary tuberosity via pterygoid plates to sphenoid bone)

Horizontal fractures from shear forces can occur at anatomically weaker regions between the following horizontal buttresses (Fig 2.2):

1. Supraorbital rim (frontal bar)
2. Infraorbital rim
3. Zygomatic arch (zygoma to temporal bone)
4. Palatine bones in continuity with the alveolar process

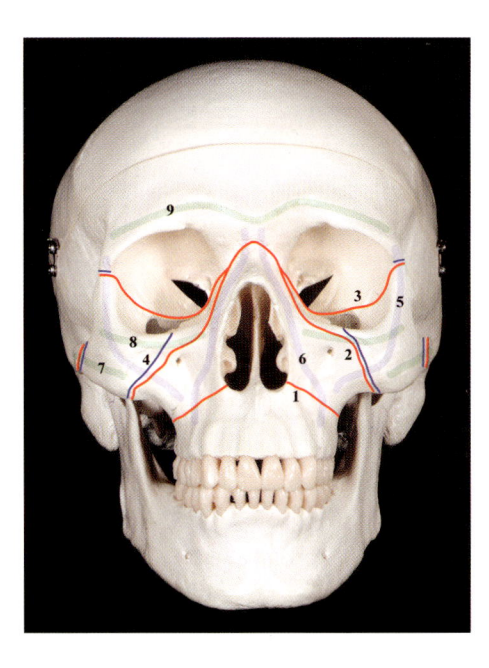

Fig 2.2. Midface buttresses and fracture patterns displayed on a skull

1. *Le Fort I fracture*
2. *Le Fort II fracture*
3. *Le Fort III fracture*
4. *Zygomatic complex fracture*
5. *Zygomatic vertical buttress*
6. *Nasofrontal vertical buttress*
7. *Zygomatic arch horizontal buttress*
8. *Infraorbital horizontal buttress*
9. *Supraorbital horizontal buttress*

Table 2.1. Classification of midfacial fractures

Midfacial fractures can be categorised as follows:	
Dento-alveolar	A fracture involving only the dento-alveolar part of the maxilla (or mandible).
Le Fort I	Horizontal fracture line separating palate from maxillary complex, running just above floor of nasal cavity (Fig 2.2).
Le Fort II	Horizontal fracture line involving antero-lateral walls of maxillary sinuses and crossing bridge of nose superiorly ('pyramidal') (Fig 2.2)
Le Fort III ('craniofacial dysjunction')	High horizontal fracture through nasofrontal buttress (involving cribriform plate therefore mechanical and infection risk to olfactory nerves and other contents of anterior cranial fossa), orbital floors and zygomaticofrontal sutures laterally (Fig 2.2).
Nasal and Naso-orbito-ethmoidal (NOE) complex fractures	Fracture pattern depends on the direction and magnitude of force. A horizontal blow may cause only a lateral shift of the nasal bones, whereas a frontal blow is more likely to result in buckling of the septum and ethmoidal involvement as the septum is driven posteriorly. NOE fractures are associated with additional frontal or anterior cranial fossa fractures and like Le Fort III injuries, you should maintain a high suspicion for intracranial injury.
Zygomatic arch and Zygomatic complex	Both may lead to flattening of the malar prominence, which can be very pronounced with a fracture of the zygomatic complex. With a zygomatic complex fracture, posterior displacement can interrupt the orbital floor leading to ocular complications (see section on orbital fractures below) (Fig 2.2)

It is important to realise that often the above fracture patterns do not occur in isolation but can occur in combination.

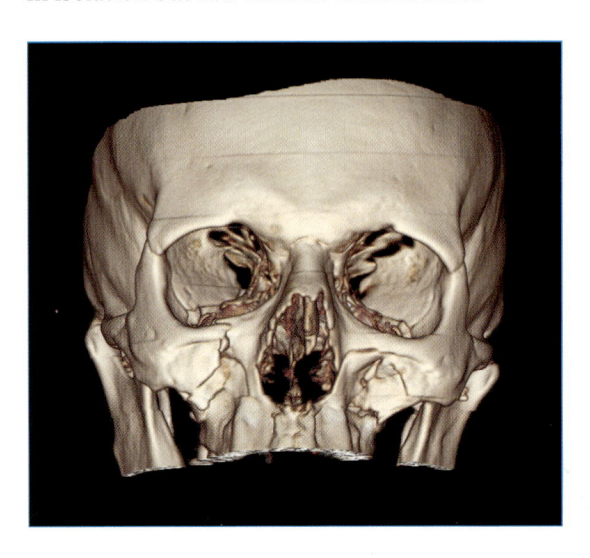

Fig 2.3. Reconstructed CT of the midface. Left Le Fort I fracture and right incomplete Le Fort II fracture

MANAGEMENT OF DENTO-ALVEOLAR FRACTURES

Fractures of the alveolus of the mandible or maxilla will be associated with dental trauma and possible displacement and/or fracture of the teeth. For management of dental trauma see page 72.

Alveolar fractures, together with the associated teeth, need to be reduced by manual reduction under LA and then stabilised using either a wire splint (see 'Tooth splinting' page 170) or, depending on the local facilities, a suck down splint may be manufactured.

MANAGEMENT OF ORBITAL FRACTURES

WHEN TO ADMIT THE PATIENT?

All orbital fractures with abnormal eye signs (e.g. blowout fractures of the orbital floor/medial wall, associated with inferior rectus entrapment or in cases of retrobulbar haemorrhage) should be discussed immediately with the on-call senior and on-call ophthalmologist for urgent review. These are highlighted in Table 2.2 below. The window of opportunity to operate upon these fractures is considered to be within 6 hours, before ischaemic muscle necrosis develops.

Table 2.2. Clinical signs indicating admission and urgent intervention in orbital fractures.

Eye signs	• Restriction of any ocular motility (in particular upwards gaze with entrapment of the inferior rectus muscle in orbital floor fractures) • Diplopia • Abnormal pupillary response to light and/or accommodation (suggesting CNII/III deficit) • Abnormal/changed visual acuity (suggesting CNII deficit)
Other signs	Oculocardiac reflex – a vagal response leading to: • Nausea and/or vomiting, • Bradycardia NB: Be aware that these signs can occur with a head injury and associated raised ICP, so ensure a serious head injury has been ruled out as well.

Any change in perception to the colour red (most sensitive clinical indicator of acute optic neuropathy), decreased vision, increase in eye pain or a suggestion of a tense globe (compared to the other eye) should be treated as suspicious of a retrobulbar haemorrhage (see 'Retrobulbar haemorrhage' page 57). These need to be treated immediately by a lateral canthotomy (see page 192).

In the meantime, the patient should be kept NBM, started on antibiotic prophylaxis, given regular neuro-obs & eye-obs, nursed head-up to minimise orbital swelling (and compression of vital structures) and instructed NOT to blow their nose.

Children are particularly at risk of extraocular muscle entrapment with orbital floor fractures. Due to the flexible nature of the bony floor, extraocular muscle (typically inferior rectus) and/or intraorbital fat are more amenable to entrapment in the flexible 'trapdoor' component of the floor leading to the clinical signs mentioned above. In a child that has no external signs of injury (ecchymosis, swelling, enopthalmos, etc) but restriction of ocular motility, the term 'white-eyed blow out fracture' is used. Have a low threshold for calling your senior if you are concerned about muscular entrapment as these cases require urgent surgical intervention.

WHEN CAN PATIENTS BE SENT HOME?

Closed orbital fractures (in adults) without eye signs and no other indication for admission can be managed as an outpatient:

- Discuss the patient with the on-call ophthalmologist.
- Arrange OMFS follow-up at 5-7 days as if needed, these patients should be treated within 2 weeks of the injury once the swelling has reduced.
- Consider oral antibiotics for up to 1 week.
- The patient should be advised to return if any deterioration in vision, swelling, head injury symptoms or any other concerns.
- Patients should avoid blowing their nose, flying in non-pressurised cabins and scuba diving, for 6 weeks.

MANAGEMENT OF NASAL BONE FRACTURES

Nasal fractures may be closed or open, and are managed accordingly:

CLOSED FRACTURE

Clinically closed minimally/moderately displaced nasal fractures can be managed as an outpatient and are best examined again one week after injury, once soft tissue swelling has subsided, to establish any need for manipulation under anaesthesia (MUA).

Grossly deformed clinically closed nasal fractures should raise suspicion of other co-existing facial fractures (e.g. NOE complex, see below). Some grossly deformed closed nasal fractures can undergo attempted reduction in the ED but this should be discussed with a senior as with NOE complex/base-of-skull involvement in the fracture, manipulation of the nasal bones may cause a CSF leak. It is also possible that a second reduction may be required once soft tissue swelling has settled anyway.

If the septum is grossly swollen and boggy to palpation (suggesting a septal haematoma), incision and drainage should be performed with a single size 11 blade incision or alternatively with a 19 gauge (white) needle and syringe (see 'Septal haematoma' page 188).

If the septum is swollen bilaterally, discuss with the on-call senior as there may be a compromise to all perichondrial blood supply (resulting in septal necrosis and a saddle deformity in the future).

Prophylactic antibiotics and/or topical antibiotics (e.g. chloramphenicol eye ointment or Naseptin® cream intranasally) may be beneficial.

OPEN FRACTURE

Clinically open nasal fractures should be:

- Dressed with a non-adherent dressing
- Admitted for a formal washout (unless you feel confident in performing this under local anaesthesia in the ED)
- Monitored with neuro-obs (if a NOE or base of skull fracture is suspected)
- If you are in any doubt, discuss with your on-call senior

MANAGEMENT OF NASO-ORBITO-ETHMOIDAL COMPLEX FRACTURES

Discuss with your on-call senior as these are associated with base-of-skull and medial orbital wall fractures. These may also be associated with overlying lacerations which may require closure.

Admit the patient for IV antibiotics, neuro-obs and keep NBM.

If a basal skull fracture is suspected (or confirmed by CSF leakage), the neurosurgical team should be informed immediately.

MANAGEMENT OF ZYGOMATIC ARCH/COMPLEX FRACTURES

Zygomatic fractures can either occur in isolation or associated with other fracture sites (orbit) in a classical 'tripod' fracture pattern (see page 113 for indications for operative intervention in zygomatic fractures).

ISOLATED ZYGOMATIC ARCH FRACTURES

If non-displaced these do not require operative intervention and can be managed as an outpatient and should be reviewed at 5–7 days once the swelling has settled.

If there is trismus (i.e. if they have restriction of mouth opening/closure through trapping of the coronoid process) the patient is likely to require surgery. If in doubt discuss with your on-call senior.

ZYGOMATIC FRACTURES INVOLVING THE ORBIT

Manage as per orbital fractures (see above).

MANAGEMENT OF LE FORT TYPE MAXILLARY FRACTURES

- Discuss immediately with the on-call senior as these fractures usually require operative intervention.
- Brain injury (commonly through a basal skull fracture) is a concern therefore these patients need neuro-obs.
- Admit for IV antibiotics, and keep the patient NBM.
- These patients can bleed and lose their airway as a result (requiring an intubation and emergency tracheostomy) so forewarn the anaesthetic team that such a patient is in the hospital. They prefer being proactive rather than reactive.
- If the orbit is involved, discuss the patient immediately with the on-call ophthalmologist and manage accordingly (see 'Orbital fractures' above).
- If a base of skull fracture is suspected, the neurosurgical team should be informed immediately. Ensure the c-spine has been formally cleared, as these injuries are often associated with significant force and place the c-spine at risk.
- Le Fort type fractures can result in significant haemorrhage. These patients frequently require postero-anterior nasal packing (see 'Nasal packing' page 180).
- Similarly, the use of intraoral bite blocks can help minimise haemorrhage through vertical compression of the fracture site (see page 46).

MANDIBLE FRACTURES

Fractures of the mandible are a common presentation to the OMFS team. Mandible fractures can occur in isolation but because of the 'U' shape of the mandible, lateral trauma often causes bilateral fractures. This is important to remember, as if you identify a fracture always examine the opposite side thoroughly. As with all fractures, to interpret and describe a fracture pattern, good anatomical knowledge is essential (Fig 1.6 and 2.4).

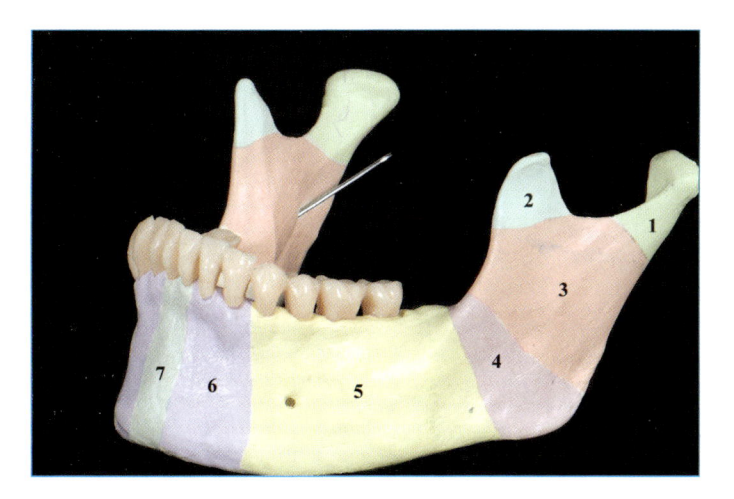

Fig 2.4. Anatomy of the mandible with regard description of fracture site

1. Condyle
2. Coronoid process
3. Ramus
4. Angle
5. Body
6. Parasymphysis
7. Symphysis

INITIAL ASSESSMENT AND MANAGEMENT

This should be as per all facial injuries (page 41).

To assess the fracture fully, you will require 2 plain radiographs at different angles to each other:

- OPG (or lateral obliques if no OPG facility)
- PA Mandible
- CT mandible may be required if the fracture is complex or the patient is unconscious

NON-OPERATIVE MANAGEMENT

If there is a single, stable, undisplaced and closed fractured then you may consider non-operative management. However, these patients need to have a stable occlusion, be compliant to attend review appointments, have good oral hygiene and tolerate a soft diet. If considering this then discuss with your on-call senior.

OPERATIVE MANAGEMENT

The mandible often fractures at 2 sites and, along with muscular displacing forces, this often makes mandible fractures unstable. Most therefore require some form of operative management, either:

- Closed reduction with IMF, or external fixation.
- Open reduction internal fixation (ORIF)

When admitting the patient prescribe the relevant medications, including antibiotics, analgesia and an appropriate mouth rinse.

CONDYLAR FRACTURES

Bilateral condylar fractures are a risk to the airway and will usually require admission and operative intervention. However, there is still some controversy regarding the management of unilateral condylar fractures. The degree of displacement and the site of the fracture will dictate the treatment options. If the patient is stable, the fracture is not displaced and there is no occlusal discrepancy, then it can be managed conservatively with a soft diet. Patients should be told to refrain from contact sports and reviewed in the outpatient trauma clinic (for indications for operative intervention see 'Unilateral Condylar fractures' page 111). If in doubt consult your on-call senior.

CONSENT

For guidelines on consenting a patient for fixation of a mandible fracture, see 'Benefits and risks of specific surgical procedures' page 144.

RETROBULBAR HAEMORRHAGE (RBH) – ACUTE ORBITAL COMPARTMENT SYNDROME

THIS IS A MAXILLOFACIAL EMERGENCY

The globe of the eye sits within the uncompressible conical bony compartment of the orbit. Therefore, pressure behind the eye, from bleeding or swelling, has no path of exit except to push the eye forwards and compress the neurovascular bundle to the eye causing an orbital compartment syndrome. Without prompt treatment, blindness will develop due to spasm of the optic blood supply and resulting ischaemia of the optic nerve.

THOSE AT RISK

- Facial fractures, notably zygomatic complex or orbital floor fractures
- Post-operative patients having undergone orbital surgery

SIGNS AND SYMPTOMS
- Loss of red vision
- Decreased visual acuity
- Tense and painful eye
- Proptosis (forward displaced eye)
- Reduced eye movement
- Fixed and dilated pupil

Patients deemed to be at risk should be monitored with eye-obs. The nursing staff must be made aware of the signs of RBH and when to notify the on-call maxillofacial team. If you suspect RBH, immediately discuss with your on-call senior and/or ophthalmology on-call. If in doubt regarding the diagnosis, orbital pressures may be measured and CT may show blood behind the globe.

IMMEDIATE MEDICAL MANAGEMENT

- Sit patient upright
- Rapid IV infusion of 100ml 20% Mannitol
- Acetazolamide 500mg IV stat and 250mg IV 6 hourly for 24 hours
- High dose IV steroid may be used e.g. 100-200mg Hydrocortisone or 8mg Dexamethasone
- Medical management should NOT delay surgical intervention, and as the OMF surgeon on-site you should be prepared to intervene surgically

SURGICAL MANAGEMENT

- Lateral canthotomy with/without decompression of muscle cone, performed in the ED or ward if necessary (see 'Lateral canthotomy' page 192)
- In post-operative patients it may be possible to reduce pressure by opening the existing incision
- Review and monitor the patient for improvement of visual acuity. If no improvement, plan for decompression/clot evacuation under GA, where appropriate.

HEAD INJURIES

INITIAL ASSESSMENT

Head injury is defined as damage to the scalp, skull or brain. This is therefore pertinent in the context of maxillofacial trauma. Head injury management depends on severity and as part of ATLS® protocol, this should be graded using the Glasgow Coma Scale (GCS, Table 2.3) where the best possible score is 15 points and the lowest possible is 3 points:

Table 2.3. Glasgow Coma Scale (GCS)

ASSESSMENT AREA	SCORE
Eye Opening (E)	
Spontaneous	4
To speech	3
To pain	2
None	1
BEST Motor Response (M)	
Obeys commands	6
Localizes pain	5
Normal flexion (withdrawal)	4
Abnormal flexion (decorticate)	3
Extension (decerebrate)	2
None (flaccid)	1
Verbal response (V)	
Orientated	5
Confused conversation	4
Inappropriate words	3
Incomprehensible sounds	2
None	1

Note: Intoxicated patients (e.g. Alcohol/Recreational drugs) should be managed as any other head injury patient. Therefore GCS deficits should be assumed to relate to head injury (rather than effects of intoxication) until proven otherwise.

GCS grading of head injury is as follows
- Mild (GCS 13-15)
- Moderate (GCS 9-12)
- Severe (GCS 8 or less)

MANAGEMENT OF HEAD INJURIES

The initial 'primary survey' should be performed by an ED senior as per ATLS® protocol. This should be followed by preliminary investigations, a comprehensive history and 'head-to-toe examination' (secondary survey).

IMPORTANT FEATURES THAT MAY SUGGEST UNDERLYING HEAD INJURY:
- Loss of consciousness (note duration and subsequent recovery)
- Amnesia (anterograde and/or retrograde)
- Headache (severity, effect of analgesia, effect of posture i.e. worse lying down or stooping)
- Visual disturbance (e.g. diplopia)
- Nausea and/or vomiting

If any of the above features are present and you are concerned that your patient may be at risk, discuss immediately with the senior ED physician or your on-call senior. Depending on the patient's history and the clinical features mentioned above, the patient may require CT scanning or admission for neuro-observation.

FACIAL LACERATIONS

GENERAL PRINCIPLES

A referral for a 'facial laceration' is not *just* a soft tissue defect but a patient who requires thorough assessment for facial trauma (see page 41) before even considering management of the wound.

When considering closure of a facial laceration under LA the following questions must be asked:

- Where is the wound and what are the functional and aesthetic implications?
- Is the wound clean or contaminated?
- Is the presentation delayed?
- Is there underlying damage to neurovascular or other important structures? Such as the parotid duct or facial nerve (see Fig 1.5b).
- Is the wound amenable to simple closure with primary sutures? i.e. is there significant tissue loss or non viable tissue?
- Does the wound require washout, exploration debridement and formal closure under GA?
- Is there an associated hard tissue injury that may require urgent operative management under GA? Therefore facial lacerations may be more appropriately managed at that time.

SPECIFIC ANATOMICAL AREAS

Some anatomical areas require particular caution, sometimes requiring exploration and formal repair in the operating theatre. If you are in any doubt, discuss the case with your on-call senior. Such areas include:

- **Eyelids.** Poor closure can have detrimental effects on corneal protection and therefore vision.
- **Lacerations near the lacrimal gland or nasolacrimal duct.** Damage to these structures risks dry eye or impaired lacrimal drainage.
- **Pre-auricular region.** The facial nerve lies within the parotid gland. Superficial branches may easily be damaged.
- **Nasal ala or columella.** Scar formation at the alar rim and columella can result in unsightly contraction deformities. If the lower lateral cartilages are involved, external valve collapse may result. In which case,

the lower lateral cartilage should be repaired (e.g. a slowly dissolvable suture such as 5/0 PDS™) before performing intranasal repair (e.g. with 5/0 Vicryl™ rapide) and extranasal repair (e.g. with 6/0 nylon).
- **Vermillion border and deep lip lacerations.** These frequently involve muscle and scar contraction can give unsightly deformities. Suboptimal repair of deep lacerations may compromise oral continence (see 'Suturing of the face and mouth' page 173).
- **Lower border of the mandible.** Be aware of the marginal mandibular branch of the facial nerve running very superficially in this region and damage can result in an ipsilateral 'smirk' deformity to the lips.
- **The neck.** See 'Penetrating neck injury' page 85.

PENETRATING AND CONTAMINATED LACERATIONS

- **Deep penetrating wounds and lacerations.** Be aware of the underlying structures that could be damaged (Fig 1.5b), especially if suggested by the history, such as a facial stabbing. Parotid duct – to assess the patency, either attempt to milk saliva from the parotid into the mouth, or intraorally cannulate the parotid duct with a plastic IV cannula sheath and inject saline while inspecting the wound for leakage. Facial nerve – assess each of the five major branches in your examination. If you suspect underlying damage to these or other important structures, discuss with your on-call senior, pack the wound and consider exploration under GA with possible microsurgical intervention.
- **Bites and contaminated lacerations.** Lacerations from bites and those sustained in dirty environments (such as sewage or rivers) carry a significant infection risk. A thorough history will elicit an approximate level of risk. All bites and suspected contaminated lacerations should be washed out thoroughly with copious amounts of sterile water/saline. For simple lacerations, primary closure is appropriate. Extensive, difficult to clean or undermined/ragged lacerations may require debridement and closure under GA. Grossly contaminated lacerations are sometimes best managed surgically in a two stage approach: the first stage involving a thorough washout with debridement as necessary and dressing, the second stage involving a 'second look' for any evidence of evolving infection (with or without delayed primary closure). Antibiotic prophylaxis should be given to cover both aerobic and anaerobic microorganisms, for example a 5–7

day course of Co-Amoxiclav, or Benzylpenicillin and Metronidazole. If in doubt discuss with the on-call microbiologist as admission for IV antibiotics may be warranted. Always check and document tetanus status (see below).

CLOSING THE LACERATION

The decision of how to close a facial laceration depends upon the size, depth and aesthetic considerations. If you do not feel confident closing the wound under LA in the ED, discuss with your on-call senior as to whether closure under GA may be more appropriate. Whilst choice of technique varies from clinician to clinician, possible options, used alone or in conjunction, include:

- Steri-strips
- Tissue glue
- Skin staples
- Sutures

For a detailed discussion of the procedure of facial laceration closure turn to 'Suturing of the face and mouth' on page 173.

ANTIBIOTIC PROPHYLAXIS

All wounds are at risk of infection. Luckily the facial soft tissues possess such a rich blood supply that serious infection is uncommon. There is much debate over the value of prophylactic antibiotics in facial soft tissue lacerations. However, some centres advise their use and a common regime would be 5–7 days of Co-Amoxiclav 625mg TDS PO, or Clindamycin 300mg QDS PO if penicillin-allergic.

TETANUS PREVENTION

All patients should have up-to-date tetanus immunity. If they have not received a vaccination within the last 10 years, a booster is often recommended and should be administered in the ED. Even if the patient's immunity is up-to-date, tetanus-prone wounds (large, contaminated, those with underlying fractures, those containing foreign bodies, those in patients suffering from systemic infection and/or delayed in presentation) warrant consideration of additional tetanus prophylaxis (intravenous tetanus immunoglobulin) and these cases should be discussed with the on-call microbiologist.

DRESSING THE WOUND

- Where feasible, it is preferable to place a non-adherent dressing such as Mepitel® or Jelonet® and cover with an overlying adhesive dressing, which aids compliance with wound care in the subsequent recovery period.
- If the adhesive dressing will not stick to the skin, try dabbing on and around the sutured wound with Benzoin Tincture (Friar's Balsam). This is antiseptic and creates a 'tackiness' which can effectively aid dressing adhesion.
- If the wound is in a hair-bearing region, fabric dressings will not adhere very easily so dress with Opsite™ spray.
- Wounds on mobile facial features can be dressed with an ointment such as 1% Chloramphenicol, applied twice daily.

WOUND CARE ADVICE

- Patients should be advised to keep the wound dressed, clean and preferably dry for long enough for epithelialisation to take place. Typically 3–5 days, after which the wound can be showered.
- Sutures on the face should typically be removed at 5 days but possibly later (7–10 days) on mobile areas or where wound closure was tighter than preferable. This can be done at the patient's GP surgery or in your outpatient department if appropriate.
- Scalp and neck sutures are typically removed at 7–10 days.
- Patients should be advised to return if there is any sign of infection (pain, swelling, warmth, redness, pus/discharge).
- Scar revision is not normally indicated until a minimum of 6 months post initial injury.

FACIAL BURNS

Due to the proximity to the airway facial burns carry potentially life-threatening complications. Therefore, these patients should be managed according to ATLS® principles and in general they are managed by burns specialists. However, with minor facial burns, you may be asked to provide initial assessment and advice on management.

FIRST AID

With heat burns or scalds, the area should immediately be run under cold water for at least 10 minutes. Chemical burns should be irrigated ideally with sterile water, never with another chemical (e.g. alkali for acidic burn) as this may cause further tissue damage through endo/exothermic reactions. If possible, take clinical photographs, they will aid review and help stop the need to remove dressing to assess the injury.

After stopping the burn process with first aid measures, dress the burn with cling-film. Do not apply lotions or ointments immediately as these will mask the burn appearance and impair clinical assessment by a burns specialist.

Contact the on-call plastic surgery team or local burns centre for further advice.

ASSESSING BURN SEVERITY

Burns can vary in severity according to:
- Total Body Surface Area (TBSA) - as a rough guide, the patient's palm equates to 1% of their TBSA. According to the 'Rule of Nines' the head and neck is 9% of TBSA.
- Depth of burn - which can be assessed as shown in the table below

Table 2.4 Classification of burn severity

Degree of burn	Sub-definition(s)	Clinical findings
First degree	Superficial	Erythema only (this is clinically not included in the TBSA involvement)
Second degree	Superficial partial thickness	Produces blistering of skin, painful.
	Mid dermal	Mottled pink colour, painful to touch, normal or brisk capillary refill
	Deep dermal	Mottled pink colour, painful to touch, sluggish capillary refill but will bleed on pricking with a fine (yellow) hypodermic needle.
Third degree	Full thickness	Painless, leathery appearance, no obvious capillary refill response, no bleeding on pricking, hair pulls easily from surface.
Fourth degree		Burn involving deeper tissues (fascia, muscle, bone)

Superficial and superficial-partial thickness burns can be managed with dressings alone and the local burns specialist may be able to provide advice on management over the telephone. However, deeper burns frequently require prompt debridement and possibly skin grafting.

EPISTAXIS

Nosebleeds may arise from a multitude of local and systemic causes, or a combination of both. Commonly, the cause is local in origin: idiopathic, inflammatory or traumatic. Alternatively, epistaxis may occur with a systemic coagulopathy (pathological or drug-induced) and/or hypertension.

MANAGEMENT

Broadly speaking, epistaxis can be anterior, posterior or both. In general, most bleeds are anterior in origin (Fig 1.8 no.13) and the bleeding point is often visible under direct visualization of the septum with a nasal speculum and good light (e.g. head-mounted lamp). However, in the OMFS patient cohort, a significant proportion will have posterior bleeds or perhaps a combination of anterior and posterior bleeding in association with midfacial fractures.

Patients with posterior epistaxis tend to have a significant amount of bleeding in the postnasal space (which can be seen at the back of the oropharynx when performing intraoral examination). These patients will not respond favourably to measures designed to deal with anterior bleeding alone. Be aware of the complications of nasal packing in patients with basal skull fractures and have a low threshold for discussing with the on-call neurosurgeon.

ANTERIOR EPISTAXIS

Anterior bleeds are usually (but not always) easier to control than posterior bleeds. If you think that the bleeding is anterior in origin, consider using the following stepwise approach:

1. Apply pressure to (squeeze, or if competent, ask the patient to squeeze) the 'fleshy' part of the nose for 15–20 minutes. This often controls minor anterior bleeds.
2. If this does not control the bleed, place a micro-sucker in the nostril to remove clots. Can you clearly see the bleeding point? If so, consider cautery with a silver nitrate-tipped stick. Note: cautery of the nasal septum should only be performed on one side as bilateral cautery may devitalise the perichondrial blood supply to the cartilaginous septum and result in a septal perforation.
3. Alternatively, electrocautery can be used but this should be performed by those with experience in this technique.

4. Alternatively, a combination of pressure and applying gauze soaked in 1:1000 adrenaline to the bleeding point may suffice.
5. If the above measures fail to promptly control the haemorrhage, pack the anterior nose using nasal tampons (e.g. Merocel®), a balloon device (e.g. Rapid Rhino®) or Bismuth Subnitrate Iodoform and Paraffin paste (BIPP) ribbon gauze (see 'Anterior nasal packing' page 180). Packs are commonly left in-situ for 12–48 hours and may warrant prophylactic antibiotics if left any longer.

After each intervention, reassess the effect of your actions to ensure that the bleeding is adequately controlled; if not, consider packing the posterior nasal space as well.

POSTERIOR EPISTAXIS

In this situation, it is impossible for you or the patient to manually apply direct pressure the bleeding point. Posterior bleeds usually require packing of the postnasal space to stop airway-threatening haemorrhage. This can be difficult to perform with BIPP gauze and this is often saved for anaesthetized patients. In the alert patient with acute posterior epistaxis, adequate packing can be achieved with a balloon device, such as a Foley urinary catheter with a small nasal tampon anteriorly or with a double-balloon device such as the Brighton balloon (see 'Posterior nasal packing' page 182).

POST EXTRACTION COMPLICATIONS

BLEEDING SOCKET

It is not uncommon for patients, particularly out of hours, to present acutely to the ED with a persistently bleeding socket after a dental extraction.

MANAGEMENT:

TAKE A HISTORY AS FOR ALL CONSULTATIONS:
- When was the extraction?
- Are they on any anti-coagulation medications? Are they on warfarin?
- If yes, coagulation studies may be indicated
- Are there any relevant medical conditions?

CONTROLLING BLEEDING:
- Ask the patient to bite down on saline soaked gauze.
- If not successful, try an adrenaline and/or tranexamic acid-soaked gauze for at least 30 minutes. This will achieve haemostasis in most cases.
- If bleeding persists you can use Surgicel® or ribbon gauze to pack the empty socket and achieve haemostasis (Fig 2.5).
- If required you can suture the mucosal soft tissue around the socket (Fig 2.6).
- If still bleeding, contact your on-call senior.

Once haemostasis is achieved the patient can be discharged and told to see their normal GDP (or to attend the clinic that performed the extraction) if bleeding recurs.

70　ON-CALL IN ORAL AND MAXILLOFACIAL SURGERY

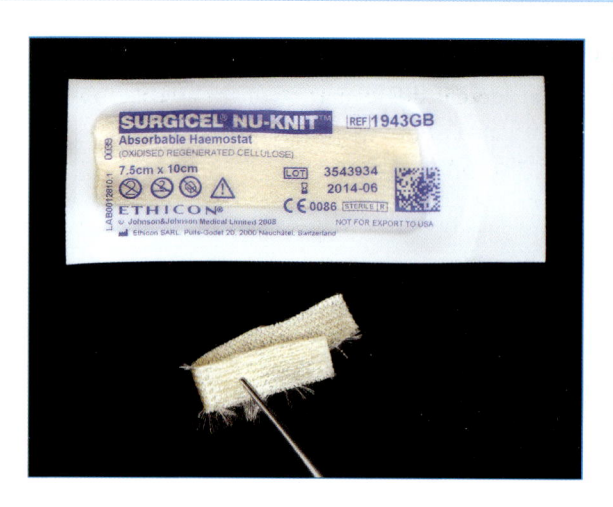

EMERGENCY DEPARTMENT

Fig 2.5. Surgicel®. Placed into the socket with non-toothed forceps.

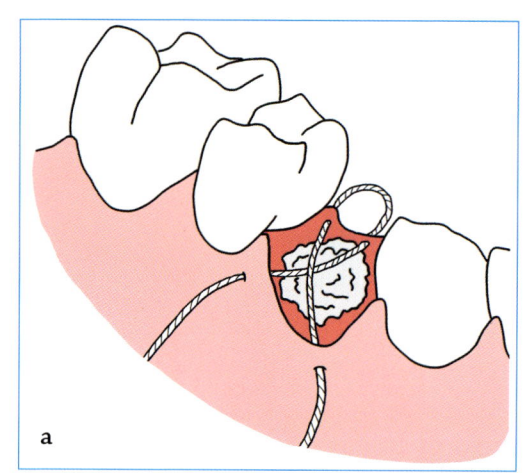

Fig 2.6. A crossed mattress suture used to close a bleeding socket. (a) Surgicel® packed into the socket of the LR4, with a crossed mattress suture placed between the gingival papillae. (b) The suture is tied to achieve haemostasis.

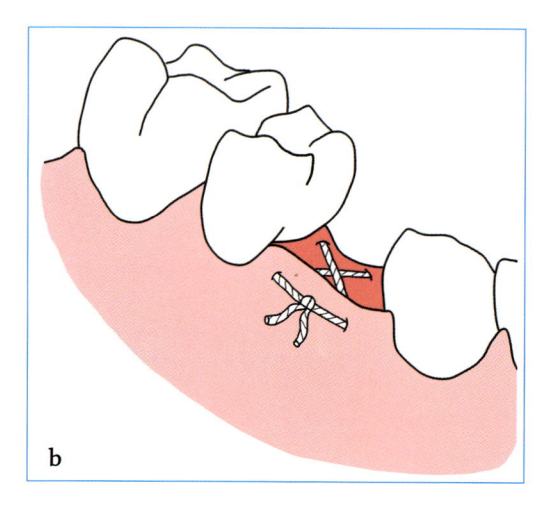

DRY SOCKET (ALVEOLAR OSTEITIS)

Dry socket is a condition where there is inflammation of the alveolar bone lining the socket after an extraction. This condition typically arises when the blood clot within the socket is lost or fails to form. The socket is exposed to the oral environment and is inflamed, but not considered to be 'infected'.

ASSESSMENT
- Patients classically present 7–10 days after extraction with an aching tooth socket.
- The patient may complain of a strange taste or halitosis.
- On inspection the socket may appear empty, partially filled with a blood clot, and/or containing debris.
- The surrounding gingiva may also appear inflamed.
- Patients who smoke or are taking the oral contraceptive pill are at an increased risk of developing this condition post-operatively.

MANAGEMENT
- Wash out and thoroughly irrigate the socket.
- Pack the socket with Alvogyl® or an appropriate alternative.
- Prescribe appropriate analgesia.
- Although controversial, if the mucosa appears inflamed, oral antibiotics can be used (commonly Metronidazole 400mg PO TDS for 3–5 days).
- Review the patient in clinic or inform them to attend their GDP or dentist that performed the extraction within 2–3 days.

DENTAL TRAUMA

The management of dental trauma is complex and differs between paediatric and adult populations, depending upon the stage of development of the tooth (see 'Eruption dates' page 16). The treatment you provide in the acute emergency setting will depend upon the dental facilities at your hospital and the dental follow-up available in the community. For up-to-date information regarding dental trauma please visit the resource www.dentaltraumaguide. org. Those that are dentally qualified will have an in-depth understanding of this topic, but for those without a dental degree the information below provides a brief overview.

Table 2.5. Dental trauma terminology

Concussion	Injury to the tooth-supporting structures but no mobility or tooth displacement
Subluxation	Injury to the tooth-supporting structures with increased mobility but no tooth displacement
Lateral luxation	Displacement of the tooth other than into or out of the socket
Intrusion	A tooth displaced further into its socket
Extrusion	A tooth partly but not completely displaced out of its socket
Avulsion	A tooth completely removed from its socket

DENTAL TRAUMA ASSESSMENT (TOOTH IN SOCKET)

As for all patients, take a detailed history. Do not focus on the tooth and ignore the rest of the face or body. Examine for other facial injury and consult the ED team if concerned regarding head injury. As a simple tool, answer the following questions to guide your management:

1. *Is the tooth mobile?*
   a. No – no urgent treatment required. Discharge with analgesia and inform to attend GDP or acute dental services.
   b. Yes – what is the degree of mobility?
      i. *Mild mobility with no displacement (subluxation)* – patient may be discharged with reassurance and no treatment. Inform patient to adhere to soft diet and attend GDP or acute dental services.

ii. *Moderate/Severe mobility and/or risk to airway* – tooth needs to be splinted (see 'Tooth splinting' page 170) or in paediatric cases extraction may be required if a primary tooth is involved. If tooth is not in-line with other teeth then treat as below and then splint.

2. *Is the tooth in line with other teeth?*
   a. *Yes* – no further treatment required.
   b. *No* – Is the tooth displaced (*lateral luxation*)? Is the tooth pushed into or out of the socket (*intrusion/extrusion*)?
      i. *Lateral luxation* – consider the possibility of a dento-alveolar fracture. In this case the tooth may be 'wedged' between two fragments of bone. Reposition (under LA) and splint with soft diet advised. Patient should attend GDP or acute dental services for follow-up. Primary teeth should be treated conservatively to avoid damage to underlying permanent tooth, refer to paediatric specialist dentist if in doubt.
      ii. *Intrusion* – Intruded primary teeth should be referred to a paediatric specialist dentist due to risk of damage to underlying permanent tooth. Immature permanent teeth (open apex) intruded <7mm can be treated conservatively, >7mm will require surgical or orthodontic repositioning. Mature permanent teeth (closed apex) intruded <3mm can be treated conservatively, >3mm will require surgical or orthodontic repositioning. If tooth is stable inform patient to attend GDP or acute dental services, if unstable consider acute repositioning and splinting.
      iii. *Extrusion* – Primary teeth extruded <3mm can be repositioned (under LA) and splinted, >3mm require extraction. Permanent teeth should be repositioned (under LA) and splinted, with soft diet advised. Patient should attend GDP or acute dental services for follow-up.

3. Is the tooth fractured?
    a. No – no further treatment required.
    b. Yes – does the fracture involve the pulp (complex dental fracture)?
        i. No – no urgent treatment required. Discharge with analgesia and inform to attend GDP or acute dental services.
        ii. Yes – bleeding may ensue and haemostasis will need to be achieved. Irrigate with sterile saline and apply a temporary dental restoration (e.g. Calcium Hydroxide, if possible) and inform to attend GDP or acute dental services.

AVULSED TOOTH (OUT OF THE SOCKET)

- If a primary tooth – **do not re-implant**.
- If a secondary tooth – re-implant and splint. When re-implanting the tooth, achieve anaesthesia with local buccal infiltration, holding the tooth by the crown – gently wash away any visible dirt and then re-implant carefully.
- If unsure – See 'eruption dates' page 16, or discuss with on-call senior.

Mostly importantly, with avulsed teeth is the extraoral drying time. This is the time the tooth is out of the socket. In the emergency setting your priority is to get the tooth back in the socket and secure it in place. The GDP or paediatric dentist can do the rest.

If you get a call about an avulsed tooth – either advise to keep the tooth in a physiological medium (milk, saline, or saliva) and attend the ED/acute dental services immediately. If clean, the tooth can be re-implanted at the scene.

TMJ DISLOCATION

TMJ dislocation is a relatively common presentation to the on-call OMFS team and may be a first presentation or as part of a cycle of recurring dislocations with/without associated joint disease. When the TMJ dislocates, the condyle lies in front of its articular eminence as shown in Fig 2.7.

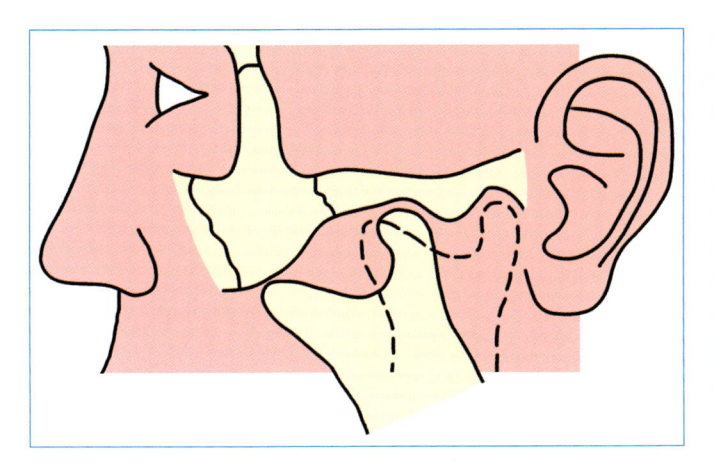

Fig 2.7. Anatomical representation of the dislocated condyle leaving the glenoid fossa to lie anterior to the articular eminence

ASSESSMENT

- When and how did it happen?
- Has the patient had similar episodes previously? If so, how was this managed?
- The patient will have an open mouth that they cannot close.
- Palpate the jaw, is there a depression in front of the ear where the condyle should be?
- The patient will likely be in pain and muscle guarding may be evident?
- Is it unilateral or bilateral?

Radiographic investigation may not be needed if an obvious dislocation. If you are in doubt about the diagnosis, an OPG or condylar views may be required.

MANAGEMENT

Manual reduction should be attempted as soon as possible. However, if you are not experienced with this, or if any complications are present, then discuss with your on-call senior.

- Give analgesia before the procedure: Nitrous oxide +/- morphine. Consider giving LA either extraorally around the TMJ or intraorally by posterior superior alveolar block
- Position the patient seated in a chair (ideally) or sat up in bed.
- Inform them what you are going to do and how you are going to do it
- Ask them not to speak or open their mouth after it is relocated for at least a minute.
- Stand in front of the patient.
- Ask for assistance from a colleague or nurse to support the patient's head and stop it tilting forward as you relocate the jaw.
- Place each of your thumbs intraorally (wrapped in gauze) resting on the retromolar region; use your fingers to grip the mandible extraorally.
- Using a 'down and back' motion, apply downwards pressure with your thumbs. You should feel the condyle 'pop' back into place.
- In patients with recurrent dislocation a barrel bandage may be useful.
- Prescribe analgesics and anti-inflammatory medications to take home.
- Encourage a soft diet for 24-48 hours.
- Instruct the patient to limit their mouth opening to prevent recurrence
- Book the patient for outpatient follow-up as appropriate
- If unsuccessful, discuss with your senior, as the patient may require muscle relaxants and/or a GA.

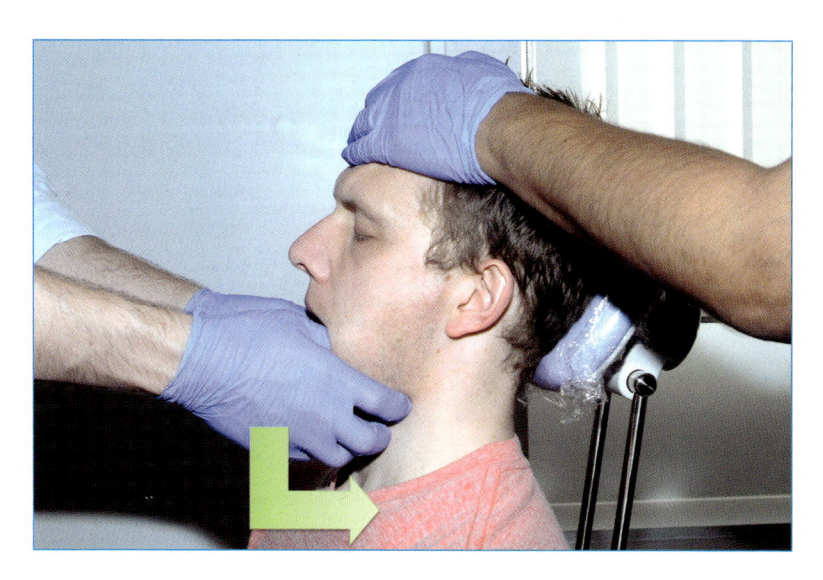

Fig 2.8. Reducing a dislocated mandible. Note support of patients head and position of hands around mandible.

OROFACIAL AND NECK SPACE INFECTIONS

Orofacial and neck space infections are commonly bacterial and often due to a dental source. They are one of the few presentations that have the potential for rapid life-threatening consequences due to the proximity of the upper airway.

The head and neck contains numerous communicating potential cervicofascial spaces through which infection can spread and collections can form (Fig 2.9).

- Sublingual space
- Submandibular space
- Buccal space
- Buccinator space
- Pterygoid space
- Lateral pharyngeal/Parapharyngeal space (consider nasoendoscopy)
- Retropharyngeal space (consider nasoendoscopy)

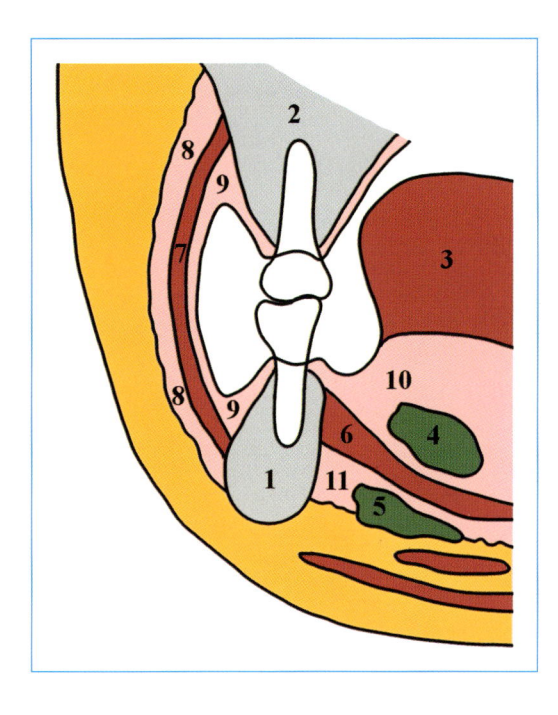

Fig 2.9. Coronal section of cheek and oral cavity to show the routes of spread of dental sepsis

1. *Mandible*
2. *Maxilla*
3. *Tongue*
4. *Sublingual gland*
5. *Submandibular gland*
6. *Mylohyoid muscle*
7. *Buccinator muscle*
8. **Buccal space**
9. **Buccal sulcus**
10. **Sublingual space/floor of mouth**
11. **Submandibular space**

HISTORY

Patients may complain of preceding dental pain, or other symptoms indicating a source of infection.

Certain patients are at higher risk of soft tissue infection:

- Diabetics
- Immunocompromised states (e.g. on chemotherapy/HIV/suffering from other systemic infections etc.)
- Soft tissue trauma/breaching of mucosal or skin barriers (e.g. insect bites/iatrogenic etc.)
- Exposure to atypical/virulent organisms (e.g. foreign travel)

EXAMINATION

In the examination, the following features should be reported both extraorally and intraorally

- Swelling (site, size, fluctuance)
- Is the FOM raised? Is the patient able to swallow saliva or instead sat forward drooling?
- Erythema and spreading cellulitis/lymphangitis (Note: mark borders of erythema with a skin marker pen to asses spread and response to treatment).
- Trismus/loss of other neuromuscular function
- Sinus at skin/mucosa
- Tenderness of teeth to percussion/palpation.
- Lymphadenopathy
- Can the lower border of the mandible be palpated

The patient may show systemic signs of infection:

- Fever (typically >37.4 degrees Celsius)
- Raised blood inflammatory markers (white cell count, C-reactive protein)
- Tachycardia

WHEN TO ADMIT PATIENTS

Can you drain the abscess/collection under LA? Does it require formal drainage and exploration under GA?

If there is a small localised collection amenable to drainage under LA in the ED, this can be performed and the patient sent home on oral antibiotics with follow-up at 48-72 hours. Large collections however require formal incision and drainage under GA. If cellulitis is present, it almost always warrants admission for IV antibiotics due to more effective tissue penetration through the IV route.

Is the patient systemically unwell?

If the patient is systemically unwell (tachycardic, pyrexial, marked leukocytosis for example) admission is required for blood cultures and empirical IV antibiotics and drainage under GA if appropriate.

IMAGING

- With very superficial collections, imaging may not be required at all.
- If a subcutaneous and/or deep collection of pus is suspected and warrants urgent incision and drainage, imaging is usually required. This can be in the form of an OPG to confirm dental pathology and identify possible teeth requiring treatment. CT or USS may help in operative planning to determine which facial space is involved and may occasionally help in image-guided drainage performed by the radiologist.
- Typically, ultrasound is the image of choice for rapid localisation of superficial soft tissue collections. A request for a skin marking should be made on the request form to aid localization of the abscess in theatre. If the radiologist is confident, relatively superficial/small abscesses can be drained at ultrasound scanning and gives a MCS sample before starting antibiotics.
- For a deep abscess/collection or investigation of possible bony involvement, CT or MRI is the gold standard investigation of choice (discuss with on-call radiologist).

TREATMENT

- LA or GA drainage if appropriate with/without dental extraction.
- Send blood cultures, pus swabs and pus samples where possible for Gram stain and MC&S
- Keep the patient NBM if going to be operated upon
- Give antipyretics and analgesics
- Consider IV fluids if the patient is dehydrated or NBM

- Prescribe antibiotics (see below)
- Nurse the patient in a head-up position
- Consider Dexamethasone (8mg IV) to reduce swelling
- For guidelines on consenting a patient for incision and drainage of an Orofacial/neck space infection, see 'Benefits and risks of specific surgical procedures' page 144.

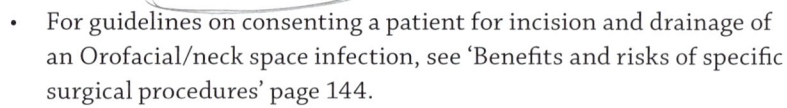

ANTIBIOTIC CHOICE

Depending on the microbial source, antibiotic choice will vary. However, patients should be started on empirical antibiotics and modified if necessary once culture/swab results are available. Always consult your Hospital Antibiotic formulary.

Co-Amoxiclav 1.2g IV TDS/625mg PO TDS

or

Benzylpenicillin 1.2g QDS + **Metronidazole** 500mg IV TDS

(the addition of Metronidazole arguably provides greater anaerobic cover)

(Clindamycin 600mg IV QDS/300mg PO QDS if penicillin allergic).

Children can be treated empirically with Co-Amoxiclav in appropriate doses (check your local or national paediatric drug formulary e.g. BNF) or alternatively discuss with the on-call microbiologist.

SPECIFIC COMPLICATIONS

SEPTIC SHOCK

If the patient shows signs of septic shock (e.g. hypotension, reduced urine output and in later stages cool peripheries/altered consciousness) treat as per the Acutely Unwell Patient section page 106.

LUDWIG'S ANGINA AND AIRWAY COMPROMISE (SEE 'LUDWIG'S ANGINA' PAGE 82)

Infections of the neck/perioral infections can threaten or compromise the patient's airway and if there is any clinical suspicion of this, contact the on-call senior and anaesthetist immediately.

ORBITAL CELLULITIS

In addition to routine antibiotics the patient will need to be seen by the ophthalmologist immediately and may require surgical exploration under GA. It is important to differentiate between preseptal and postseptal infections. Postseptal infections are associated with limited and/or painful ocular motility and proptosis and require urgent treatment.

NECROTISING FASCIITIS

Any patient with necrotic-looking superficial tissues, palpable surgical emphysema (subcutaneous crepitus) or severe pain on palpation should be discussed immediately with the on-call senior and microbiologist in case of a life-threatening necrotizing fasciitis. Soft tissue radiographs and/or CT scan should be taken to look for evidence of gas-forming organisms.

INTRACRANIAL COMPLICATIONS

Intraoral and facial infections can lead to cavernous sinus thrombosis or a brain abscess and these should be considered in anybody with altered neurological signs on examination. These are emergencies and should be discussed with the on-call senior and neurosurgeon immediately.

LUDWIG'S ANGINA

This is an acute floor of mouth cellulitis which can lead to a bilateral infection of the submental and submandibular spaces. The commonest source of infection is from a lower 3rd molar and organisms involved are usually anaerobic. The resulting tissue oedema and swelling poses a **significant airway risk**. If Ludwig's angina is suspected, contact the on-call senior immediately as early intervention minimises this complication.

CLINICAL FEATURES
- Cellulitis (may not be visible) of the external neck/under the chin
- Painful swelling/oedema of neck which is tender to palpation
- Pyrexia and signs of systemic inflammatory response (elevated white cell count/CRP)
- There may be a palpable tender lymphadenopathy, but tissue oedema may mask this
- Mouth opening may be limited and the tongue may be pushed up by the floor of mouth swelling
- Patients may be sat forward and drooling
- If the patient has any signs of airway obstruction (see box below) this is an emergency. Contact the on-call anaesthetist immediately.

Signs of impending airway obstruction
- Raised floor of mouth
- Drooling
- Difficulty swallowing
- Hoarse voice
- Visible stenosis/oedema on flexible nasoendoscopy

MANAGEMENT
- Use ABCDE approach, paying close attention to ensuring the airway is patent and that the patient is fluid resuscitated to prevent septic shock from developing.
- Contact on-call senior +/- anaesthetist immediately.
- Book and consent for surgery for formal incision, exploration and drainage +/- tracheostomy.
- Arrange for a post-operative ITU/HDU bed.

ACUTE SIALADENITIS

This describes an acute inflammation of the salivary glands. It typically affects the parotid glands although can affect the submandibular and rarely the sublingual glands. It is usually bacterial in origin.

CLINICAL FEATURES
- A painful swelling which arises over the gland
- Overlying skin erythema
- Tenderness on palpation of the gland
- Pain worse on eating and drinking
- Turbid saliva expressed on palpation/massage of the gland
- Cervical lymphadenopathy

MANAGEMENT

The majority of patients can be managed in the outpatient setting:
- Give analgesia
- Swab of discharge from duct
- Massage the gland to encourage the release of pus and saliva
- Broad-spectrum antibiotics

If systemically unwell, manage as for severe orofacial/neck infections:
- Appropriate fluid rehydration and IV antibiotics
- Imaging, if required to confirm diagnosis in the form of USS. Avoid sialography because of the risk of developing bacteraemia
- If abscess present or develops then book for theatre for incision and drainage under GA

INFECTED SEBACEOUS CYST

A sebaceous or epidermoid cyst is often found in hair-bearing areas of the body. They typically occur on the scalp, scrotum, neck, shoulders and back, although can also occur on the face and other non hair-bearing regions. They can vary in size from a few millimetres to several centimetres. Histologically they are comprised of keratinous debris lined by keratinising squamous epithelium and are associated with hair follicles.

They can often persist but remain asymptomatic for many years. However, if they require treatment, in order to prevent recurrence, the entire cyst and its contents should be removed with an ellipse of skin which typically centres on the small punctum present over the cyst. Recurrence is common if even a small portion of the lining is left in situ.

CLINICAL FEATURES

In the on-call setting these typically present with an acute infection:

- History of previous painless lump, now acutely painful
- Warm, tender, erythematous, fluctuant mass
- Punctum visible

MANAGEMENT

- The resulting abscess will often require drainage under LA, if feasible this can be done in the ED (see 'Draining a Sebaceous cyst' page 184).
- If there is evidence of superficial cellulitis, a 3-5 day course of an anti-staphylococcal oral antibiotic (e.g. Flucloxacillin 250-500mg QDS) can be given.
- The cyst may need to be excised 4-6 weeks later, once the initial infection has resolved, to prevent further episodes.

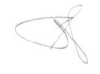

PENETRATING NECK INJURY

A penetrating neck injury is defined as any wound, which extends deep to platysma. Because of the vital underlying structures, these injuries can have devastating effects. As such, they should be managed as per ATLS® protocol. There will be multi-disciplinary input within the ED, and you should involve your on-call senior. Neck trauma is described as per the zone of injury (see Fig 1.14)

MANAGEMENT
- Early assessment by the anaesthetic team is mandatory and patients may require endotracheal/nasotracheal intubation or tracheostomy.
- Patients should be nursed in a supine position to limit the risk of air emboli.
- Haemorrhage control should be achieved with direct pressure rather than blind clamping if possible.
- Wounds should not be heavily probed for fear of dislodging formed clot leading to recurrent bleeding.
- It is important to remember that there is a risk of subclavian vein injury in zone 1 trauma, so fluids should run in the contralateral arm to avoid the risk of extravasation in these patients.

Patients with 'hard' signs are typically managed with immediate exploration in the operating theatre. Hard signs include:

- Severe active bleeding
- Large expanding haematoma
- Unresponsive hypovolemic shock

Other associated injuries are shown in Table 2.6.

Table 2.6. Clinical signs of associated penetrating neck injuries

Group	Signs	Notes
Airway injuries	Respiratory distress, stridor, hoarseness, Subcutaneous emphysema.	As per the ATLS® protocol, the airway requires immediate intervention
Nerve injuries	Cranial nerve deficit or hemiparesis	May not require operative intervention if patient otherwise stable
Oesophageal injuries	Bleeding from oesophagus, leakage of saliva, subcutaneous emphysema or these may be asymptomatic.	May lead to neck or mediastinal abscess formation
Vascular injury	Active haemorrhage, expanding haematoma, vascular bruit and diminished or no pulse.	Likely to need urgent intervention

In the event of a symptomatic but haemodynamically-stable patient, there may be scope for urgent CT angiography prior to exploration, particularly in zone 1 or 3 injuries.

If patients are asymptomatic, then they can be assessed using CT angiography, endoscopy, bronchoscopy and swallow studies. Those that have positive findings are explored in theatre. Those with negative findings can often be conservatively managed under close observation.

BLEEDING AND ULCERATED GUMS

Occasionally a patient may present to the ED with acutely bleeding or ulcerated painful gums. The most common cause for this is a severe form of gum disease (gingivitis, see below). However, when taking the history you should screen for causes of bleeding such as anticoagulant medication and clotting disorders. Bleeding can be managed with local measures as detailed in 'Bleeding socket' page 69. For painful oral ulceration, Difflam® mouthwash is a useful adjunct. If local measures do not achieve haemostasis discuss with your on-call senior or the ED/medical team if bleeding is linked to an underlying medical condition.

ACUTE NECROTISING ULCERATIVE GINGIVITIS (ANUG)

ANUG is an infection of the gingival tissues. It is commoner in the younger population, typically between the ages of 10 and 30 years. It is thought to occur in patients with a reduced host defence and as such is associated with smoking, stress, immunocompromise or malnutrition.

CLINICAL FEATURES

- Painful, inflamed and bleeding gums
- Inflammation starting at the interdental papillae and spreading along the gingival margin.
- Gingivae may become ulcerated, leading to 'punched out' necrotic lesions.
- Patients may complain of halitosis or a 'bad taste' in the mouth.

MANAGEMENT

- Analgesia
- Mouth rinse – Chlorhexidine
- Antibiotics – PO Metronidazole 200–400mg TDS for 3–5 days
- Patients should be instructed to attend a dentist as soon as possible for further treatment.

WARD

PRESCRIBING INTRAVENOUS FLUIDS

You will be called to give IV fluids in a variety of scenarios for a variety of reasons, such as the peri-operative period or in those acutely unwell requiring fluid resuscitation. It should not be forgotten that all IV fluid regimes need careful consideration and planning.

WATER REQUIREMENTS

As a guide an unstressed healthy adult requires **30-40ml/kg/day**.

For an average male of 70kg that equates to approximately **2.1-2.8 L/day**.

ELECTROLYTE REQUIREMENTS

When prescribing fluids your primary electrolyte concerns are sodium and potassium:

Na^+ 2mmol/kg/day

K^+ 1mmol/kg/day

Obviously the above figures will rise or fall depending on the patient's age and individual medical status. Your decision to start fluids and what fluids to give should be based on a combination of clinical and biochemical evidence. Always check a patient's recent biochemistry results before initiating fluid therapy.

INTRAVENOUS FLUID PRODUCTS

Fluids are described as being either crystalloid or colloid. Crystalloid fluids contain electrolytes, whereas colloid fluids contain high molecular weight molecules to mimic the colloid osmotic effect of large plasma proteins (albumin).

Because of their colloid osmotic pressure, colloids have been favoured in resuscitation of shocked patients (acute hypovolaemia), although recent evidence shows no difference between crystalloid and colloid resuscitation. For correcting electrolyte imbalance and fluid maintenance, crystalloids are the fluid of choice.

SO HOW MUCH FLUID SHOULD I PRESCRIBE?

Commonly patients will just require 1-2 bags of IV fluid peri-operatively to keep them hydrated. For prolonged periods, patients require carefully prescribed fluid maintenance regimes.

NORMAL FLUID MAINTENANCE

The regimes below are based on an average 70kg adult. Your regime can be adapted accordingly to account for these patient factors.

REGIMEN A:

- 1L Normal Saline 0.9%   over 8hours   plus 20mmol K+
- 1L 5% Dextrose   over 8 hours   plus 20mmol K+
- 1L 5% Dextrose   over 8 hours   plus 20mmol K+

TOTAL = 3000ml with 154mmol Na+ and 60mmol K+

(So called 'one salty, two sweet' regimen)

REGIMEN B:

- 1L Dextrose-Saline   over 8 hours   plus 20mmol K+
- 1L Dextrose-Saline   over 8 hours   plus 20mmol K+
- 1L Dextrose-Saline   over 8 hours   plus 20mmol K+

TOTAL= 3000ml with 90mmol Na+ and 60mmol K+

Give high dose potassium fluids with caution as there is a risk of arrhythmias. Use a maximum dose of 40mmol.L at a maximum rate of 20mmol/hour. If in doubt consult your on-call senior or medical team.

FLUID MAINTENANCE IN CHILDREN

Fluid maintenance in children is dependent upon their weight. The 24-hour fluid requirement for a child up to 50kgs is calculated using the following formula:

100ml/kg for first 10kg

50ml/kg for the next 10kg

20ml/kg for each remaining kg

5% Dextrose - 0.45% saline is normally the fluid of choice (consult paediatrician if in doubt).

e.g. for a 23 kg child.

Fluid requirements = (100 x 10) + (50 x 10) + (20 x 3) = 1560ml/24 hours

PATIENTS WITH ALTERED FLUID/ELECTROLYTE REQUIREMENTS

It is more common for OMFS patients to require more as opposed to less IV fluids. Dehydration post-operatively is a common complaint and patients who have suffered trauma or have an on-going infection are at an increased risk. It is an easily treatable condition, but one that carries a profound risk of morbidity should it escalate to acute kidney injury (acute renal failure).

CLINICAL SIGNS OF DEHYDRATION
- Dry mucous membranes
- Increased skin turgor
- Decreased urine output – Normal urine output = >30ml/hour

BIOCHEMICAL ABNORMALITIES OF DEHYDRATION
- Raised Urea
- Raised Creatinine
- Raised Haematocrit
- Raised Albumin

If the insult upon the kidneys is severe then the patient can be classified as having acute kidney injury (AKI). While AKI is graded 1 to 3 based upon severity, you only need to be able to recognise if a patient's blood creatinine rises 1.5-2 fold (150%-200%) from baseline, or their urine output drops to <0.5mg/kg/hour for 6 hours (generally less than 30ml/hour) as these findings indicate AKI and should be assessed and managed promptly to prevent further deterioration.

CAUSES OF ACUTE KIDNEY INJURY

The best way to view AKI diagnostically is to consider: Is it a **Pre-renal** cause (*something happening before the kidneys*), a **Renal** cause (*the kidneys are the problem*), or a **Post-renal** cause (*something happening after the kidneys*)?

- **Pre-renal:** Acute volume depletion – bleeding, dehydration, hypotension. *This is most common in surgical patients.*
- **Renal:** Acute tubular necrosis, nephrotoxic induced, vascular origin.
- **Post-renal:** Obstruction of urinary flow – calculi, cancer, blocked catheter.

ASSESSMENT AND MANAGEMENT

You assess the patient as you would do for any acutely sick patient, but if you follow the 'DONUT' acronym then you can't go wrong!

D – DEHYDRATION:

Optimise the IV fluids. Be aggressive i.e. 1 hour (1 litre) bag, 4 hour bag, etc. Be cautious in the elderly and patients with heart failure (see below). These patients may need input from the hospital physician/'medical team'.

O – OBSTRUCTION:

Catheterise the patient to monitor urine output. Get a bladder scan and USS to rule out a post-renal cause.

N- NEPHROTOXINS:

Review their medications and stop any other possible offending drugs. Don't forget that NSAIDs and ACE-inhibitors are nephrotoxic.

U – URINE:

Get a urine dipstick, and send off for MC&S.
- *Infection* – white cells and nitrites
- *Pre-renal cause* – dip NAD
- *Renal cause* – Blood and Protein
- *Post-renal cause* – Blood

T – THINK:

What is the underlying cause?

If you can get this far and have stabilised the patient and treated the common causes for AKI then you have done well. If in doubt call the medical team for further input.

Table 3.1: Patient factors influencing fluid and potassium requirements

When patients require increased fluid
• Infection, sepsis, fever
• Increased GI losses, vomiting or diarrhoea, intestinal fistulae
• High losses from surgical drains
• Dehydration post-operatively, with or without intraoperative blood loss
• Shock (see 'Acute Patient Management' section, page $$)
When patients require fluid restriction
• Pulmonary oedema secondary to heart/renal failure
• Hepatic failure with ascites
• Obvious fluid overload
• Elderly patients at risk of fluid overload
When patients require increased potassium
• Vomiting and diarrhoea
• Intestinal fistulae
• Drugs – diuretics
• Endocrine disorders – Cushing's, Conn's Syndrome
• Alkalosis for other reason
When patients require potassium restriction
• Renal failure
• Drugs – K+ sparing diuretics, ACE inhibitors
• Previous large blood transfusion
• Endocrine disorders – Addison's disease
• Metabolic Acidosis

GLUCOSE CONTROL

HYPOGLYCAEMIA

This is a common presentation, that is both easy to treat but easy to forget, hence the phrase 'ABC – **DEFG**, *Don't Ever Forget Glucose*' recounted on all resuscitation courses.

Many of the patients you will see as the on-call OMF surgeon are at risk of hypoglycaemia:

- Diabetics – especially insulin controlled diabetics or those on sulphonylurea oral medication
- Elderly patients
- Patients with infection e.g. dental sepsis
- Patients under the influence of alcohol or other drugs
- Patients having undergone periods of starvation either pre or post-operatively

Table 3.2. Clinical presentation of hypoglycaemia

Glucose < 3.5	Sympathetic overactivity	*Tachycardia, palpitations, anxiety, tremor, sweating*
Glucose < 2.5	Neuroglycopaenia	*Confusion, slurred speech, focal neurological deficit (mimics a stroke)*
Glucose < 1.5	Hypoglycaemic coma	*Unconsciousness*

MANAGEMENT:

Treat the patient according to the 'Acutely unwell patient' section, page 106. Seek senior or medical help if in doubt.

PATIENT ALERT AND ABLE TO SWALLOW:

- Oral glucose e.g. Glucogel®, Lucozade.
- Also give them a long acting carbohydrate such as toast.
- Re-assess patient.

PATIENT UNWELL/COMA OR UNABLE TO SWALLOW:

- 25-50ml of 50% IV Glucose/Dextrose with a saline flush (through a large peripheral vein)

- If no IV access, give 1mg IM Glucagon.
- Reassess patient, continue to monitor blood glucose levels, repeat if necessary.

HYPERGLYCAEMIA

Glucose persistently > 12mmol/L

In all patients with diabetes, acute illness or recent surgery, an increase in counter-regulatory 'stress' hormones opposes the action of insulin and leads to a deterioration of glycaemic control. The most important diagnosis in patients with elevated blood glucose is to exclude diabetic ketoacidosis (DKA) or hyperosmolar non-ketotic coma (HONC). In patients with a persistently high glucose always consult your senior or the medical/endocrine team.

WHAT TO DO WITH DIABETICS BEFORE SURGERY

The combination of pre-operative fasting and the hormonal stress response experienced during surgery makes diabetic patients vulnerable to episodes of poor glycaemic control. Therefore, try to put any diabetic patient first/early on the operating list.

The points below are guidance only and your hospital should have formal guidelines regarding pre-operative management of diabetic patients. Always inform the anaesthetist of the patient's diabetic status and if in doubt discuss with the anaesthetist at the time of the pre-operative assessment.

GENERAL POINTS

- Metformin should be stopped 48hrs before a GA, as it can precipitate a metabolic acidosis.
- Blood glucose should be monitored 4 hourly (pre and post-operatively).
- If a patient remains NBM for a prolonged period of time (i.e. delayed surgery) or if the blood glucose rises (>12-15mmols/L) start a variable rate insulin infusion (sliding scale).

MINOR SURGERY

- Patient on oral medication only – continue normal regimen.
- Patient on insulin therapy – omit the pre-operative dose of insulin. Restart insulin once the patient resumes an oral diet.

MAJOR SURGERY

- Patient on oral medication only – omit pre-operative dose of medication on day of surgery. Longer acting oral medications may need to be omitted on the evening prior to surgery.
- Patient on insulin therapy – omit the morning dose of insulin and start a variable rate insulin infusion once the patient is nil by mouth (for restarting insulin see below). For patients on long acting insulin preparations, consider giving a reduced dose (50-75%) the day before surgery.

EMERGENCY SURGERY

- Start variable rate intravenous insulin infusion. Be aware of ketoacidosis risk if glucose levels rise. *Consult on-call anaesthetist if in doubt.*

VARIABLE RATE INTRAVENOUS INSULIN INFUSION (SLIDING SCALE)

These are simply an infusion of insulin and fluid adjusted to take into account the patient's blood glucose levels. They typically use a continuous infusion of 8 hourly 5% Dextrose with 20mmol/L K$^+$, together with a short-acting Insulin (e.g. Actrapid®). The blood glucose is measured every hour and the insulin dose increased or decreased accordingly. *N.B Always consult your local hospital guidelines.*

STOPPING THE VARIABLE RATE INTRAVENOUS INSULIN INFUSION

Post-operatively the infusion must be continued until the patient is eating normally and has resumed their normal insulin therapy.

- Allow the patient to eat 2 full meals.
- Patients on fast acting insulin – stop the infusion 1 hour after the first dose of normal insulin therapy.
- Patients on long acting insulin – stop the infusion 4 hours after the first dose of normal insulin therapy.
- N.B If in doubt consult your medical/endocrine team or diabetic nurse specialist

TRACHEOSTOMIES

TRACHEOSTOMY TUBES

Patients you will encounter with tracheostomies include:
- Head and neck oncology patients.
- Patients with airway-compromising facial trauma or infection.
- Patients undergoing elective tracheostomies for prolonged weaning off ventilation in ITU.

In the immediate post-operative period patients will likely be on ITU/HDU, but when they move back to the ward you will be called to deal with tracheostomy problems. An understanding of the components and types of tracheostomy tubes, and how to deal with their complications is essential.

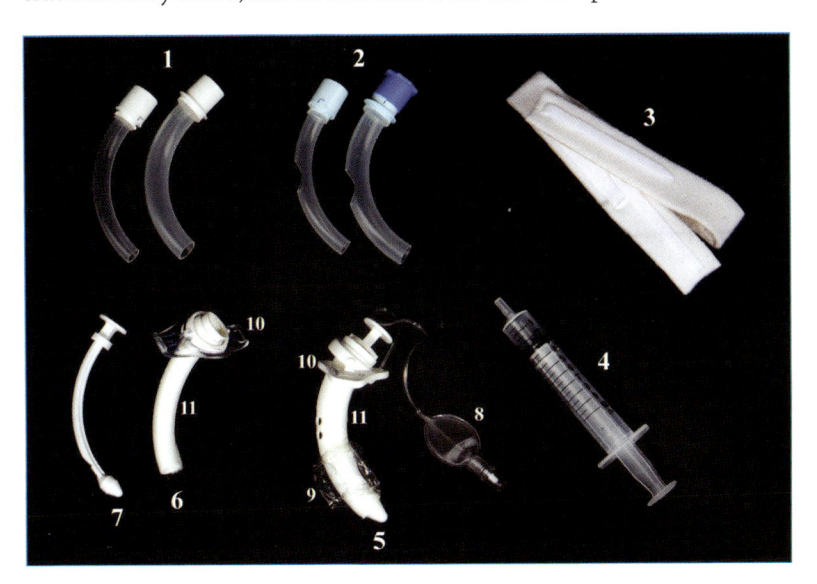

Fig 3.1. Assortment of tracheostomy tubes and components

1. *Non-fenestrated inner tubes (size 7.5 and 9.0)*
2. *Fenestrated inner tubes (size 7.5 and 9.0)*
3. *Neck tie*
4. *10ml syringe for cuff inflation*
5. *Cuffed tracheostomy tube, outer cannula with obturator in-situ (size 9.0)*
6. *Non-cuffed tracheostomy tube, outer cannula (size 7.5)*
7. *Obturator*
8. *Pilot balloon (demonstrates cuff inflation)*
9. *Inflatable cuff*
10. *Neck plate/flange*
11. *Shaft*

TYPES OF TRACHEOSTOMY TUBES:

- *Cuffed and non-cuffed tubes* – The inflatable cuff on a tracheostomy tube allows it to sit firmly in the trachea and form a good air seal.
- *Fenestrated and non-fenestrated tubes* – The fenestration (a hole in the wall of the tracheostomy tube) allows air to pass up and over the vocal cords allowing the patient to speak. The drawback of this is that saliva can enter the tube and pass into the lungs.

Take the time to familiarise yourself with the tracheostomy tubes used in your hospital. Be able to inflate the cuff, perform suction, and change the inner tube and entire tracheostomy tube if required.

TRACHEOSTOMY CARE

THINGS TO REMEMBER

- Do not over-inflate the cuff, this can cause damage to the tracheal wall and cause stenosis
- To avoid tube displacement, make sure the tracheostomy tube is kept in place with tape, and/or a neck tie and/or sutured in place (but check local practice – some surgeons do not want neck ties if they have just completed a microvascular anastomosis)
- Ensure regular tracheal suction and saline nebulisers
- Prescribe humidified oxygen
- Oral suction may be beneficial, paying careful attention to any tissue flap in-situ
- Keep a spare tracheostomy tube and tracheal dilators next to the patient in case of tube displacement or other emergency
- Refer for chest physiotherapy

BE AWARE OF THE POST-OPERATIVE COMPLICATIONS OF A TRACHEOSTOMY

- Infection at the tracheostomy site
- Displacement of tube out of stoma (and difficulty with reinsertion)
- Bleeding; this can be potentially serious if the tracheostomy tube erodes through the posterior wall of the trachea
- Recurrent laryngeal nerve injury
- Chest infection

DISTRESSED TRACHEOSTOMY PATIENT

You may be called to see a patient with a tracheostomy who is in distress. This will be because of displacement or obstruction of the tube. This may be indicated by the following features:

- Persistent air leak, not abolished by inflating the cuff
- Unable to ventilate or an increase in ventilation pressures
- Hypoxia or cyanosis, with obvious difficulty breathing

MANAGEMENT

Manage according to the ABCDE approach:

- Start high flow oxygen
- If the patient is in obvious distress with airway compromise call for help immediately. Either from your on-call senior if they are on-site, or the on-call anaesthetist.
- Remove the inner tube to check if it has become occluded.
- Use a suction catheter to check for an occlusion and or remove any debris
- A flexible nasoendoscope may be useful to directly visualise the trachea
- If necessary the tracheostomy tube can be replaced with a temporary smaller tube. If you are unfamiliar with this procedure then you will need to call your senior. You will need tracheal dilators and/or Langenbeck retractors and a good light source.
- If the tracheostomy tube is completely dislodged and the patient has no patent airway you will need to replace the tube as soon as possible. This may require the use of retractors and a willing assistant. If the surgeon has placed rescue sutures, by gently pulling on these it will help expose the tracheostomy window in the tracheal wall.

FLAPS IN ORAL AND MAXILLOFACIAL RECONSTRUCTION

In reconstructive surgery, a flap is tissue transferred from a donor site to recipient site with its associated blood supply. Flaps can be broadly classified according to tissue type, blood supply or anatomical donor site. A graft differs in that the tissue's blood supply is not transferred with it.

FLAP CLASSIFICATION

TISSUE TYPE

- Can be a single tissue type (skin, fat, fascia, muscle, bone)
- Can be a composite of any of the above tissues (e.g. fasciocutaneous, adipofascial, myocutaneous, osseocutaneous)

BLOOD SUPPLY

- Random pattern: blood supply is derived from a non-specific artery/network of unnamed vessels). Commonly a small local flap.
- Axial: flap with a named blood supply running along its axis in a variety of configurations

CONTIGUITY OF DONOR AND RECIPIENT SITE

- A flap transferred from a donor to immediately adjacent recipient site is a local flap
- A flap transferred to a non-adjacent region is a distant flap, and can be subdivided into:
    a. Pedicled flap (the blood supply remains sourced from the donor site)
    b. Free flap (the blood supply is disconnected at the donor site and anastomosed to vasculature at the recipient site using microsurgical techniques)

SHAPE/ORIENTATION OF FLAP

- Commonly used to describe local flap subtypes. e.g. Limberg (rhomboid) flap

FLAP MONITORING

Distant pedicle and free flaps require regular monitoring post-operatively, typically for at least 72 hours. In the first 24 hours, the flap is typically checked hourly, and even more frequently in the first few hours post-operatively (as per the surgeon's preference). Flap failure rates continue to reduce but are still a major complication in head and neck reconstructive surgery. Flap failure usually occurs within 72 hours of surgery and usually relates to either a problem of flap perfusion (i.e. ischaemia), or venous drainage (i.e. congestion).

Table 3.3. Flap Assessment

Temperature
• Warmth is a sign of good tissue perfusion. Be concerned if the flap is cooler than adjacent recipient site tissues.
Capillary refill
• Is it normal? (1-2 seconds)
• Is it brisk? This suggests venous congestion
• Is it delayed? This suggests inadequate arterial perfusion
Turgor
• Some degree of turgor is expected with any inflammatory insult on the tissues such as surgery but is the flap different to native recipient site tissue?
• Is the flap firm and/or swollen? This could indicate congestion or an underlying haematoma which compresses its vascular pedicle, further exacerbating any impairment in arterial perfusion or venous drainage
Colour
• Is the colour normal? Remember the donor site skin may be physiologically different in appearance to the recipient site.
• Ecchymosis may reflect an underlying haematoma.
• A pink flap is generally healthy providing all of the above factors are normal, otherwise it could be congested
• A pale flap suggests impending ischaemia
Doppler ultrasound signal
• Commonly used by some surgeons to grossly demonstrate arterial inflow. Gently place the Doppler probe on the flap with jelly usually at a marker suture/ink mark and check for an audible arterial waveform.
Pin-prick testing
• Perform with caution and discuss this with your senior before undertaking. In many units, this is a test that is done only be the on-call consultant.

IDENTIFYING THE CAUSE OF A FAILING FLAP

Table 3.4. Causes of a failing flap

Local causes

Impaired arterial inflow/perfusion or venous drainage can be affected by:
• Compression of the pedicle:
   a. Intrinsic (haematoma, tissue oedema, 'kinked' pedicle from incorrect orientation of pedicle vessels intraoperatively). This will require an immediate return to theatre.
   b. Extrinsic (tight dressings, tightly closed wounds, pressure points, incorrect neck positioning causing 'kinking' of pedicle) dressings should be loosened, sutures may need to be removed, the patient may be repositioned, haematoma drained.
• Thrombosis/embolism (arterial or venous). This commonly requires a return to theatre but in some centres, thrombolysis has been used. May relate to local factors (anastomosis) or systemic (hypercoagulable states).

Systemic causes
• Hypovolaemia (inadequate arterial inflow to flap) • Hypoxia (could be secondary to post-operative atelectasis or pulmonary oedema). • Hypercoagulability (see above). • Coagulopathy (leading to bleeding complications of hypovolaemia and haematoma formation and pedicle compression). • Other systemic disease. • Smoking (nicotine causes vasospasm and could theoretically compromise flap perfusion). • Iatrogenic (use of vasopressors should take into account the risk to flap perfusion). • Temperature (a warm patient makes a warm flap – if the patient is cold, consider a Bair Hugger™).

ENTERAL FEEDING

This is a method of delivering food directly into the stomach/duodenum/jejunum, bypassing the oral cavity.

There are several indications, but in OMFS the principle indications are patients recovering from major head and neck surgery who are unable to swallow and protect their airway and sedated patients requiring long-term nutrition.

ROUTES OF ENTERAL FEEDING:

NASOGASTRIC (NG) TUBE

- Often the first choice in instituting enteral feeding in the acute setting.
- It is a temporary measure and can be used for up to 1 month before a long-term option is required

PERCUTANEOUS GASTROSTOMY

- Indicated when long-term enteral feeding is required (>1 month) but in the absence of gastric pathology
- Commonly available routes of insertion include: Open surgical gastrostomy, percutaneous endoscopic gastrostomy (PEG) – minimally invasive surgical combined with endoscopic technique (the most common method) or radiologically inserted gastrostomy (RIG) – an alternative for patients who cannot tolerate endoscopy

NASOJEJUNAL (NJ) TUBE

- This is used when the feed needs to be delivered further down the GI tract for practical or safety reasons (to feed distal to operative sites, prevent gastro-oesophageal reflux and subsequent aspiration pneumonia)

POST-INSERTION CHECKS AND DAILY CARE

NG/NJ TUBE:

After the feeding tube is inserted, it is essential to check the position of the tube to ensure that the feed can be delivered safely (i.e. not into the airway and down the right main bronchus). These checks include:

- pH testing with universal indicator paper (the pH should be <5.5)
- Chest radiograph to check that the end of the tube is below the diaphragm and appears to be in the region of the stomach/jejunum

PEG/RIG:

Check the post procedural instructions from the person who inserted the tube. Often RIG tubes have a retentive 'button' device, which needs to be removed after a few days (if left can cause gastric ulceration and perforation).

Check your local protocol with regards to when feeding can be commenced. The patient's dietician should be able to advise on this. Often a period of time is required post-insertion to ensure no complications arise (peritonitis, etc.) and a regime of 'water only' feeding may be required at first.

DAILY CARE

- Gastrostomy/Jejunostomy sites should be checked daily for signs of infection (pus/cellulitis), ulceration and displacement
- With NG/NJ tubes, the nostrils should be checked daily for internal and external pressure ulcers
- Feeding tubes should be flushed before and after use to prevent blockage
- Gastric aspirates should be measured regularly to ensure adequate gastric emptying after feeding. Gastric outlet obstruction or delayed emptying could predispose the patient to reflux and aspiration pneumonia.

COMPLICATIONS OF ENTERAL FEEDING

There are numerous risks for patients undergoing procedures for enteral feeding while some complications may arise after the patient's return to the ward:

LOCAL

- Bleeding – Either intraabdominal or at the wound site
- Infection/Ulceration – At the percutaneous insertion site or in mucosal areas leading to rhinitis/sinusitis/pharyngitis/oesophagitis/gastritis etc.
- Damage to other intraabdominal structures at percutaneous insertion
- Tube misplacement
- Leak of feed/gastric perforation/peritonitis
- Feed aspiration in patients with gastro-oesophageal reflux. Therefore patients should be fed with a head-up tilt of 30-45 degrees.

SYSTEMIC

- Gastroenteritis +/- septicaemia, from bacterial contamination of feed
- Diarrhoea/constipation
- **Refeeding syndrome**
    - Sudden institution of enteral feeding after a prolonged period of starvation exerts a physiological stress on the body
    - A relatively high carbohydrate load institutes osmotic fluid shifts and a surge in insulin release, resulting in an acute loss of electrolyte homeostasis. This can lead to confusion, arrhythmias and even seizures.
    - Patients are particularly at risk of hypophosphataemia, hypokalaemia and hypomagnesaemia. Therefore re-institution of feeding should be slow, dietician supervision is useful and electrolytes should be monitored very closely (daily biochemistry, magnesium and calcium at least).

EVALUATING THE ACUTELY 'UNWELL' PATIENT

As with all acute medical presentations, the assessment and management of the acutely unwell patient on the ward is best achieved using an 'ABCDE' approach. While this book is unable to provide a comprehensive discussion of all acute medical and surgical conditions, below we provide a basic framework for assessing an 'unwell' patient. If you can get through this first, instigate initial management and have the information to hand when you call for help this will save valuable time.

Often a severely unwell patient is described as 'shocked'. Physiologically the term **'shock'** relates to *'an abnormality of the circulatory system that results in inadequate organ perfusion and tissue oxygenation'*. Signs of shock include:

- Tachycardia (heart rate>100 beats/minute),
- Hypotension (systolic blood pressure <100mmHg)
- Tachypnoea (respiratory rate> 20 breaths/minute)
- Decreased urine output
- Altered mental status

In OMFS the common acute scenarios are **septic shock** e.g. secondary to dental sepsis, or **hypovolaemic shock** e.g. secondary to haemorrhage in facial fractures. Therefore, the knowledge to recognise these and treat accordingly is essential. For example, a shocked patient who is pyrexic and peripherally warm and vasodilated may have septic shock, in contrast to the cold peripherally vasoconstricted patient in hypovolaemic shock. While beyond the scope of this book, take the time to familiarise yourself with the other types of shock that may require specialist care, including **anaphylactic**, **cardiogenic**, **obstructive** and **neurogenic shock**.

AIRWAY

Is the airway patent? Are there upper airway noises or stridor? Does the patient look visibly short of breath?

Give Oxygen – 15L/min through a non-rebreathable mask

Is the patient conscious enough to maintain his or her own airway? If you feel that their upper airway is at risk an immediate resuscitation (crash team) call is warranted. In the meantime take a stepwise approach to improve and maintain the airway:

1. Airway manoeuvre: Chin lift – head tilt (not if suspected cervical spine injury) or jaw thrust

2. Airway adjunct: If the airway continues to remain compromised, consider an airway adjunct such as a Guedel oropharyngeal airway or a nasopharyngeal airway (not if suspected basal skull injury or patient has undergone skull-base surgery)
3. Semi-definitive airway: If the patient's condition fails to improve consider a laryngeal mask airway (LMA™)
4. Definitive airway: this is performed by the anaesthetist (intubation)

BREATHING
- Inspect and palpate the chest for expansion. Percuss for hyperresonance or dullness.
- Auscultate for breath sounds in all zones: superior, middle and inferior zones bilaterally. *Can you hear crackles? Are there decreased or absent breath sounds?*
- Assess the respiratory rate and oxygen saturation
- Any of the above abnormalities should be further investigated based on your clinical findings, for example requesting a chest radiograph or obtaining arterial blood gas analysis

CIRCULATION
- Assess heart rate, blood pressure and urine output (normal >30ml/hr). Obtain an ECG if cardiac symptoms or tachycardia are present
- Obtain the patients temperature. Pyrexia (>37.4 degrees Celsius) may indicate 'sepsis' or 'septic shock'. Consider PO/IV antibiotics. If the cause of infection is unclear, screen for common sources of infection (chest – CXR, urine – urine dip, bowels – stool sample)
- Gain IV access. While doing so take blood and send for analysis – Full blood count, Urea and Electrolytes, Coagulation studies, CRP, etc.
- If the patient has signs of shock, after gaining IV access, give a fluid challenge of either crystalloid or colloid (see page 89)
- The volume of fluid to be given depends on the degree of hypovolaemia which can be estimated by the adversity of the patient's observations/urine output etc. A 500ml fluid bolus is acceptable in a young healthy person, after which the response should be assessed and the bolus can be repeated.
- Be cautious of giving large (>500ml) boluses of fluid in frail/elderly/malnourished patients or those with a history of cardiac failure as this can precipitate acute cardiac failure and pulmonary oedema

DISABILITY

- Assess the patient's level of neurological disability: this may be affected by airway, breathing, circulation or other causes (e.g. hypoglycaemia, sedatives, analgesics, electrolyte disturbance etc.). This is most accurately assessed and recorded by the Glasgow Coma Score (GCS) (see 'Head Injuries' page 59).
- Any patient with acute cognitive impairment should be closely monitored with neuro-observations for any further deterioration
- A fingerpick blood glucose should be measured immediately as hypoglycaemia is a common and reversible but potentially fatal cause of impaired consciousness
- If the cause of decreased consciousness is not immediately obvious and reversible (overuse of opioids/sedatives), contact the on-call senior for further advice

EXPOSURE

Examine the patient for any bleeding. Such as epistaxis, neck swelling, blood in the oropharynx. Look at the patient as a whole (not just the head and neck), are there any other clinical signs to explain the patient's deterioration? For example: Is the patient warm or peripherally under perfused? Is there bleeding from operative sites? Are there any rashes associated with anaphylaxis or meningococcal sepsis?

Once an intervention is made (e.g. giving IV fluids and antibiotics) the patient should be reassessed to monitor an improvement. If the condition is not improving seek senior help early.

THE NEXT STEP

- The ABCDE approach is a good way to assess and manage a patient with immediate effect. However, it is not particularly thorough so after assessing these basics, conduct a thorough but focused history and systems examination and check all available charts and observations.
- Senior input may be required from your team or another specialty to further manage the patient
- If however, you are happy that the patient is stable, continue with routine care

ON-CALL IN ORAL AND MAXILLOFACIAL SURGERY

PATIENTS ON WARFARIN

Warfarin has an essential role in prevention of thromboembolic stroke in patients with atrial fibrillation and prevention of thrombus formation in mechanical heart valves. It also forms the mainstay of long-term treatment for previous venous thromboembolic events.

The level of the anticoagulant effect of warfarin within a patient is assessed using the INR (international normalised ratio, derived from the prothrombin time). Patients with atrial fibrillation and those on prophylaxis due to a previous pulmonary embolism or deep vein thrombosis require a typical INR range of 2-3, while patients with metallic heart valves require a typical INR range of 3-4.

WARFARIN DOSING

Warfarin dosing is not an exact science and varies hugely between patients, relating to variability in pharmacokinetics and pharmacodynamics. Warfarin is a vitamin K antagonist and its effect is heavily dependent on hepatic metabolism.

Patients who need special consideration when prescribing warfarin:
- Hepatic impairment
- Renal impairment
- Pregnancy
- Breast feeding
- Elderly frail patients (the starting dose can be decreased. i.e. from 10mg to 8mg or 5mg)

For starting/restarting patients on warfarin consult your local hospital protocol. If a patients INR rises above their target range consider omitting 1-2 doses then rechecking the INR.

REVERSAL OF WARFARIN

Reversal of warfarin in situations of haemorrhage can be achieved with vitamin K and blood products. Always refer to your hospital protocols first and if in doubt discuss with the on-call haematologist.
- If minor haemorrhage give Vitamin K 1-3 mg oral/IV.
- If major haemorrhage with a high INR, give vitamin K 5mg IV and consider prothrombin complex concentrate or fresh frozen plasma.

WHAT TO DO WITH PATIENTS ON WARFARIN PRE-OPERATIVELY

Decisions regarding warfarin dosing pre-operatively will depend on the indication for its use, the peri-operative risk of thromboembolism and the type of surgery being performed. For example a patient with atrial fibrillation and no previous thromboembolic events may be considered 'low risk', a patient with atrial fibrillation but previous thromboembolic events when not anti-coagulated would be 'moderate risk', and a patient with a metal heart valve would be 'high risk'. However, it should be noted that this is a grey area and if in doubt always consult the physician managing the patient's condition.

- **Minor surgery** – Patients undergoing minor surgical procedures such as dental extractions or skin surgery can continue taking their warfarin peri-operatively, with a check INR the night before/morning of surgery
- **Major surgery with low risk patient for thromboembolism** – Stop warfarin 5 days before surgery and check INR night before/morning of surgery
- **Major surgery with moderate risk patient for thromboembolism** – Stop warfarin 5 days before surgery. Start prophylactic dose low molecular weight heparin (e.g. 40mg enoxaparin SC) 4 days before surgery. Stop heparin morning of surgery.
- **Major surgery with high risk patient for thromboembolism** – Stop warfarin 5 days before surgery. Start therapeutic dose low molecular weight heparin (e.g. enoxaparin 1.5mg/kg SC) 4 days before surgery. These patients may need to be started on IV unfractionated heparin the night before surgery for better peri-operative bleeding control.

Accepted INR levels to perform major surgical procedures are commonly <1.8-2 although surgeon preference and procedure bleeding risk are major factors. Levels for minor surgery varies considerably and if the INR is outside the normal target range then surgery may need to be delayed.

Generally speaking, warfarin can be restarted the evening/morning after surgery. However, patients at risk of thromboembolism will need further post-operative heparin until the INR is within therapeutic range.

CLINIC

ACUTE TRAUMA CLINIC

Patients are commonly referred to the trauma clinic having been initially assessed in the ED, or at another hospital. Such clinics are suitable for the review of patients where immediate surgical management is not appropriate, and the decision on whether to operate or not is often deferred whilst waiting for bruising and swelling to settle. However, deciding in the ED setting which patient can be reviewed in a deferred manner and who needs to be seen urgently can be difficult, especially if there is diagnostic doubt regarding the presence of a fracture on imaging.

The type and site of the fracture/injury will dictate when patients should be seen in the trauma clinic.

Common injuries that are deferred for maxillofacial trauma clinic review include the following:

- Unilateral condylar fractures (with no malocclusion)
- Zygomatic arch fractures
- Zygomatic complex fractures
- Orbital floor fractures (without evidence of muscular entrapment)
- Anchored disc phenomenon (acute closed lock)

FOR ALL PATIENTS ATTENDING THE TRAUMA CLINIC

- Confirm the history
- Re-examine the patient with particular focus on the site of injury
- Review all available imaging

UNILATERAL CONDYLAR FRACTURES (WITH NO MALOCCLUSION)

- Ask patients how they are coping with the soft diet, and ensure they understand what a soft diet entails.
- Ensure the occlusion is even and stable. If not, surgical intervention in the form of arch bars or Leonard buttons may be more appropriate in order to re-establish a stable occlusion. In some cases, ORIF of the condyle may be considered.
- Review the radiographs and ensure the condylar fracture is appropriate for non-surgical management.

Individual surgeons will vary in how actively they wish to manage a unilateral fractured condyle but it is important to check if there is any suggestion of a malocclusion, as early surgical intervention will be the only way to correct this.

There is much debate over the suitable criteria for ORIF of the mandibular condyle. However, the following indications have become increasingly popular amongst UK OMF surgeons:

- Fracture-dislocation of the condyle
- More than 10° of angulation from the normal position
- More than 2mm overlap of the condyle and mandibular ramus.

ORBITAL FLOOR FRACTURES

These are often the most difficult fractures to diagnose and are often missed. In patients without abnormal eye signs, it is preferable to review patients in the trauma clinic 5–7 days after the injury, to allow any swelling to subside.

Full imaging, orthoptic assessment and ophthalmic review are mandatory before any surgical intervention can be arranged. The orthoptic assessment generates a HESS chart, which allows the diagnosis of ocular motility/binocular single vision defects (Fig 4.1). It measures the deviation and the amount of restriction and compensation of the ocular muscles. It is a repeatable and reliable record of orbital motility and is therefore a good way to show improvement or deterioration of any ophthalmoplegia. It is useful for those with diplopia and helps decide when not to treat an orbital floor fracture in the absence of acute eye signs. It also allows the clinician to distinguish between oedema and entrapment of the ocular muscles.

Not every orbital floor fracture requires surgical intervention, but some cases may have a delayed deformity/disability thereby requiring on-going review. In the interim, patients should be warned not to cough/sneeze/blow their nose, counselled about surgical emphysema and dystopia becoming evident once residual swelling settles.

In patients referred to the trauma clinic, typical indications for treatment of an orbital floor fracture include

- Restriction of ocular motility
- Non resolving diplopia
- Enophthalmos (either early or late)
- Hypoglobus
- As part of other midfacial fracture management (especially involving the zygomatic complex).

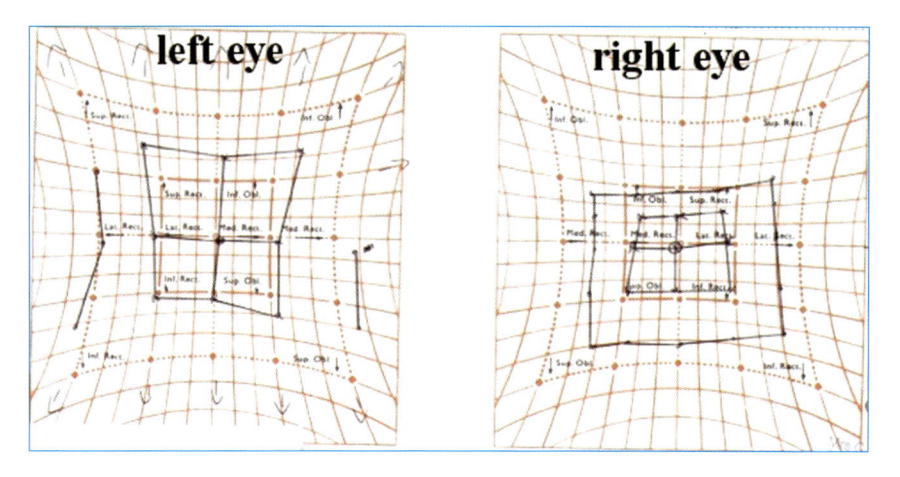

Fig 4.1. A Hess Chart: A patient with a right orbital floor fracture with restriction of upward gaze on the right side.

Early management may be preferable to delayed management, but ultimately timing will be dictated by the presence of the other injuries and the attending surgeon's preference.

ZYGOMATIC ARCH/COMPLEX FRACTURES

These fractures are often managed in a deferred fashion. However, if indicated operative management should be undertaken within 14 days.

In the instance of a zygomatic complex fracture there may be a concomitant orbital floor fracture. If the patient has not been assessed by the ophthalmic team, a formal review should be arranged as soon as possible (see previous section 'Orbital floor fractures').

Indications to fix these fractures are either:
- Aesthetics – if there is obvious flattening of the cheek concerning the patient.
- Function – if there is restricted mouth opening (because of the arch fracture impinging upon the coronoid process of the mandible).
- Vision – for management of diplopia secondary to ocular motility defect in associated orbital fractures.

ANCHORED DISC PHENOMENON (ACUTE CLOSED LOCK)

In the case of anchored disc phenomenon, there will often be a history of trauma and associated TMJ-related pain. It is often due to an intraarticular haematoma formation and fractures are often not seen on imaging. On examination there will be an open bite on the side of the trauma and a decreased MIO.

Review on the trauma clinic is required to assess for persistent symptoms and the need for any surgical intervention. The treatment of choice is arthrocentesis. This is particularly useful in those with an MIO of less than 20mm and/or a strong suspicion of an intraarticular haematoma.

ONCOLOGY CLINIC

Head and Neck oncology MDT clinics usually occur once a week. Surgical, pathology, radiotherapy and oncology staff will be present as well as speech and language therapists (SALT), dietitians and head and neck specialist nurses. The surgical disciplines of OMFS, ENT and Plastic surgery who partake in the definitive management of such patients will be involved in the surgical discussion.

All patients who undergo an oncological procedure will be reviewed on a post-operative clinic. This is usually the specialist MDT clinic but depending on local practice may be within a general clinic. As a general rule, these patients have had significant surgery and should be discussed with a senior in most instances. When reviewing these complex patients, clear concise clinical notes are mandatory. The MDT outcome sheet is a valuable source of information and should be reviewed at each appointment. It will summarise the MDT's rationale behind the patient's treatment, in addition to the patient's response to treatment.

It is important to assess and document the following information:

- Primary diagnosis
- Presence of risk factors such as smoking and HPV
- Primary management
- Histology
- Agreed follow up
- Subsequent interval scans (especially when management was essentially non surgical with chemo-radiotherapy or neck sparing).

FIRST CLINIC REVIEW POST SURGERY

Considerations here need to be centred on how the patient is coping now they are home. The patient's weight should be recorded and reviewed at every visit. It is important to assess how patients are tolerating any nutritional supplementation such as PEG or RIG feeding. Some feeding regimes may require adjustment because of bloating or diarrhoea. Some patients will complain of reflux, especially when PEG fed for tongue base tumours. Close liaison with dietitians may allow the best combination of feeding regime and medications such as prokinetic drugs (e.g. metoclopramide) or proton pump inhibitors (e.g. omeprazole).

Many patients can struggle with communication post-operatively. This is especially so with free flap reconstruction, where there may be significant swelling and oedema around the flap, which can compromise good articulation. The SALT team are invaluable in supporting patients to improve and regain their speech and swallowing function. Many SALT units can now provide tablet computer devices to help patients communicate during this process.

The surgical site needs to be thoroughly reviewed. If a peri-operative tracheostomy was placed, check that the wound is closed and healing. Check neck dissection scars are healing and that there are no retained sutures. Ask about any accessory nerve weakness (difficulty raising arms or shrugging shoulders) and test this formally. If present, early outpatient physiotherapy and advice can be useful. On-going physiotherapy support may well be required in the form of passive and active exercises after latissimus dorsi, scapula, serratus anterior and fibula free flaps, as well as orthotic boots if ankle pain or instability exists post fibula flap harvest.

Intraoral examination should centre on checking whether the oral cavity is suitably clean to ensure no wound breakdown is occurring. If patients remain nil by mouth post surgery, this makes this process easier, but soft tissue toilet may still be difficult. If any bony resection has occurred, is this surgical site covered and healing appropriately? This is essential if patients are due to have post-operative radiotherapy, as this may well need to be delayed if there are concerns.

If a histological specimen was taken during the procedure, this appointment may also be the first opportunity at which definitive histology may be available. Decisions regarding the need for further surgery or adjunctive treatment such as radiotherapy may need to be discussed, but this is usually carried out by the consultant surgeon after discussion with the MDT.

Ensure patients have telephone numbers for the Head and Neck Oncology nurse, and are made aware that should there be any concern, they should be calling in for advice. Patients who have undergone major head and neck surgery should be seen by the responsible team if they have any concerns.

In addition, some patients may have had elective dental clearances as part of their treatment. You should not assume that their own GDP is able to provide subsequent treatment. With many of these patients now being seen in designated centres, utilisation of the restorative dentistry team is usually mandatory. The GP/GDP needs to be copied into this communication so that fluoride supplements and mouthwashes, oral sprays can be added to repeat prescriptions.

Patients who complain of trismus post surgery may benefit from jaw exercises. Devices such as TheraBite® appliances, if available, can be a valuable self-support adjunct.

As with all patients, remember the role of providing support regarding smoking cessation and reinforce why they should stop/stay abstinent especially when radiotherapy has been proposed, as this is known to reduce survival and local control.

SUBSEQUENT CLINICAL REVIEWS

Provided there are no complications, as a general rule, these patients should subsequently be reviewed:

- Every month for the first year
- Every two months for the second year
- Every three months for the third year
- Every four months for the fourth year
- Every six months for the fifth year
- Until 5 years have elapsed at which stage they can be discharged.

At these review appointments:

- Review the history and how they have managed since the previous review.
- Review MDT documentation to ensure no aspect of management has been neglected.
- Conduct a thorough extraoral and intraoral examination, in particular any new intraoral mucosal changes as these may be appropriate to biopsy. As well as a general examination, focus specifically on the previous tumour site and regional lymph nodes for any signs of recurrence.
- Any history of swelling or wound breakdown should not be dismissed and requires discussion with the lead clinician as this may well be an initial sign of clinical recurrence or wound breakdown as a result of osteoradionecrosis post radiotherapy.
- Examine the donor site if a free flap reconstruction was performed.
- If they are PEG-fed, routinely the PEG site should be examined, and consideration given to when the PEG tube might need changing. If they are managing intake without PEG supplementation, then refer them for its removal.
- Do not ignore the dentition and if oral hygiene or caries management is sub-optimal, consider referring to any local facilities that may be available, or liaise with their GDP.

- If they are a year post surgery and radiotherapy, and plans have been provisionally discussed regarding definitive oral rehabilitation with the restorative team (using implants or new prostheses), remember to refer them.

PALLIATION

Some patients in the head and neck cancer clinic will not be appropriate for surgical intervention while others may not have responded to treatment or may suffer recurrences that are not amenable to further treatment. The decision against surgery is often a difficult one to make and as such these decisions are made in conjunction with the MDT.

Patients undergoing palliative therapy may often complain of symptoms including wound breakdown, fungation, wound odour, excessive secretions and pain, as well as suffering aspiration or bleeding at the tumour site.

After reviewing the MDT documentation, consider liaising with the tissue viability nurse to help with issues such as wound breakdown and fungation. There are many options to reduce odour and inflammation, which can be distressing aspects for the patient. Consider the use of metronidazole gel, Aquacel® or other topical agents to help with this. Where rapid fungation of tumour has occurred, the MDT may decide that that radiotherapy input for palliation is appropriate.

Other options that offer some symptomatic relief may include diverting nutrition so more is per PEG than mouth therefore reducing saliva secretions. This is normally performed with dietitian input.

Pain is often difficult to control in these circumstances. In addition to the analgesia suggested on the WHO pain ladder (see page 37), these patients may require many other adjuncts such as anxiolytics and neuropathic pain agents. The oncology team from the MDT will be actively involved, and input from the pain specialists may often be required.

Palliative patients may present to the on-call OMF surgeon via the ED with complications such as aspiration or a significant bleed. Therefore, clear documentation regarding acceptable input and the ceiling of care is essential.

SALIVARY GLAND CLINIC

Many patients who present to a designated salivary gland clinic will fall into one of two categories:

- They have obstructive symptoms from one or more glands
- They have a palpable lump in the region of a salivary gland

As with any other condition, careful history taking and a thorough clinical examination is mandatory.

THE OBSTRUCTED PATIENT

It is unusual to see these patients acutely on clinic, as often they will have had an episode or repeated episode of infection (see 'Acute Sialadenitis' page 83), which has been managed by their GDP, GP or the on-call OMF surgeon in the ED. Sialolithiasis (salivary stone) occurs most commonly in the submandibular gland.

ASSESSMENT

- The classical history may be present of painful swelling which occurs after mealtimes, which spontaneously resolves. It may have been a single episode or recurrent.
- Examination should involve bimanual palpation of the submandibular gland to establish whether any stone can be located.
- One should also give consideration to whether any decrease in salivary flow rate is observed compared to the other side, along with a comment as to the nature of the exudate (does it look like clear saliva or is it pus?).

INVESTIGATIONS

- OPG or a lower standard occlusal film may visualise any obvious stone as the majority are radiopaque and will be seen on plain imaging. It is important to remember that some stones however may be radiolucent.
- Ultrasound scans may demonstrate integrity of the gland, the gland architecture and the presence of any dilatation of the main duct.

If both these investigations yield no positive findings, and the history has been ratified, then the next stage would be a sialogram. However this investigation may not always be available. It relies on the patient remaining still for approximately one hour for the test to be performed so requires patient compliance. Where sialograms cannot be undertaken, CT scans may be appropriate if the index of suspicion is high enough to justify the radiation dose.

Once these results are all available, a definitive decision can be made regarding management. Stones up to 5mm in size are thought to have the potential to spontaneously deliver into the oral cavity. The duct is narrowest at the exit point, and often the stone is palpated there and is amenable to excision under local anaesthesia.

Other surgical options include basket retrieval, lithotripsy, transductal excision and excision of the gland in part or its entirety if there is evidence of chronic sialadenitis and scarring within the gland. In specialist centres, ductal dilatation, endoscopic retrieval, laser ablation or lithotripsy can all be offered as viable treatment options.

LUMP WITHIN A SALIVARY GLAND

Patients can be referred with a slow growing lump, commonly within either the parotid or submandibular gland. Depending on the referrer, the patient may be referred routinely or on a rapid access pathway as a suspected cancer. Irrespective of the mode of referral, there tends to be a degree of heightened anxiety about a lump found either by the patient themselves or their clinician, and this should be borne in mind when assessing them.

ASSESSMENT

The most likely diagnosis for such a lump in the parotid is a pleomorphic adenoma. Submandibular and sublingual lumps have a higher risk of malignancy than parotid masses. Assessment involves a through history and examination with attention to the mass itself (whether it is firm/mobile/uniform in size and its exact location).

Other differentials for such a lesion can include a Warthin's Tumour, monomorphic adenoma, lymphoma or adenoid cystic carcinoma/mucoepidermoid carcinoma, acinic cell or squamous cell carcinoma.

Local arrangements may allow this patient to attend a 'one-stop' clinic where clinical examination is followed by an ultrasound-guided FNA and imaging if required using either CT or MRI. If not, these investigations should be arranged. Once the results are available, the patient should be reviewed, the diagnosis explained and the management should be agreed upon.

MANAGEMENT

Treatment could include surgical excision of the lump itself, excision of part of the involved gland (extracapsular dissection) or the removal of the gland in its entirety, with or without radiotherapy, depending on what the definitive diagnosis is.

POST-OPERATIVE REVIEW

Post-operatively, these patients attend for yearly review for up to 5 years. They should also be asked about Frey's Syndrome (also known as gustatory sweating) for which Botox® therapy may be offered after doing a starch iodine test. They should be examined for the presence of any salivary fistulae. Also, at each visit, patients who have undergone parotid surgery should be asked about facial nerve dysfunction, which can be documented and described using the House-Brackmann scale (Table 4.1).

Table 4.1. House-Brackmann scale for grading facial nerve dysfunction

Grade	Description	Measurement	Function %
I	Normal	8/8	100
II	Slight	7/8	76–99
III	Moderate	5/8–6/8	51–75
IV	Moderately severe	3/8–4/8	26–50
V	Severe	1/8–2/8	1–25
VI	Total	0/8	0

This assessment is scored based on the upward movement of the midpoint of the eyebrow and the outward movement of the angle of the mouth. Each fixed point scores 1 for every 0.25cm of movement seen (to a maximum of 1cm). Both scores are added together to give a total score out of 8.

After 5 years the patient is discharged back to the care of the GDP/GP, who is asked to monitor them for a further 5 years.

FACIAL SKIN LESIONS

Facial skin lesions can present as areas of abnormal discolouration, lumps or ulcers. While a detailed explanation of all these lesions lies beyond the scope of this book, it is important to have a basic understanding of some of the more common lesions and more importantly be aware of suspicious lesions so if they are encountered, you can ensure they are managed promptly and appropriately. Table 4.2 outlines the lesions you should be aware of.

Table 4.2. Facial skin lesions

Name	Description	Benign/ Malignant	Management
Basal cell carcinoma	Commonest skin cancer. Slow growing with local spread. Ranges from reddish patch to pearly nodules with rolled border, telangiectasia and central ulceration.	Malignant	Should be referred to local skin cancer clinic. May require histological confirmation of diagnosis. Treatment options include excision, radiotherapy or Mohs surgery.
Capillary haemangioma	Red, lumpy area typically found around the orbit. Rapid growth in infancy with regression later.	Benign	Often spontaneously regress. Otherwise may be suitable for laser removal, embolisation or surgical excision.
Dermatofibroma	Raised swelling on skin associated with chronic trauma.	Benign	
Keratocanthoma	Dome-shaped, symmetrical lump with central plug of keratin and debris. Grows quickly for a few weeks with spontaneous resolution over 6 months.	Benign	May resolve spontaneously over many months. Can be removed by curettage, or by surgical excision.

Name	Description	Benign/ Malignant	Management
Lentigo maligna	The very earliest stage of melanoma. Slow growing lesion in sun exposed area. Typically presents as long-standing discoloured patch of skin.	Pre-malignant (for melanoma)	Urgent referral to skin cancer clinic for surgical excision.
Malignant Melanoma	Pigmented lesion with potential for metastasis. Nodular, irregular in shape, raised with colour variation	Malignant	Requires urgent referral to appropriate skin cancer clinic via rapid referral pathway.
Meibomian cyst	Retention cyst of meibomian gland which open behind the eye lashes. Obstruction of gland duct leads to stagnation of secretions and a firm, painless, round lump in tarsal plate.	Benign	Usually resolves spontaneously with warm compresses or gentle massage. May require surgical curettage or steroid injections. If becomes infected, then should be treated with topical antibiotics.
Naevus	Skin moles, typically darker than surrounding skin.	Benign	Monitor for change.
Seborrhoeic keratosis	Often occurs in elderly. May itch or catch on clothing. Appear as yellow/brown raised lump.	Benign	Often require no treatment but cryotherapy or curettage may be indicated.
Skin tags	Pedunculated small skin lump.	Benign	Observation with cryotherapy or excision if needed.

Name	Description	Benign/ Malignant	Management
Actinic/Solar keratosis	Sun-damaged skin with a highly variable appearance, ranging from rough skin to raised, warty lesions.	Pre-malignant (for SCC)	May resolve spontaneously with responsible sun protection. May require histological confirmation prior to definitive treatment (photodynamic therapy, cryotherapy, surgical excision or curettage).
Squamous cell carcinoma	Often occurs on sun damaged areas of face e.g. lips and ears. Variable appearance: red plaque, raised edges, commonly ulcerates and bleeds.	Malignant	Urgent referral to skin cancer MDT for biopsy and treatment (surgical excision, Mohs surgery or cryotherapy) +/- chemoradiotherapy.

ORAL SOFT TISSUE LESIONS

There are many different lesions of the oral cavity that will be referred to the OMFS clinic. While it is outside the scope of this book to discuss them all, a group of more common presentations are discussed below.

RECURRENT APHTHOUS ULCERATION (STOMATITIS)

Recurrent aphthous ulcers can affect up to 25% of the population. Often the aetiology remains unclear, but nutritional deficiencies and a familial predisposition have been noted.

ASSESSMENT

A careful history of these lesions is essential and should include:

- Size of ulcers
- Site of ulcers
- Number at any one time
- Time for a single ulcer to resolve
- Time between ulcer outbreaks
- Any prodromal symptoms?
- Any obvious association? (e.g. pre-menstrual or stress)
- Any systemic dysfunction? (in particular bowel or haematological)
- Presence of any scarring

> Aphthous ulceration can be classified into the following:
> - *Minor* – (most common) Ulcers <10mm with an oval shape and grey base with erythematous border. They last 1–2 weeks with no scarring.
> - *Major* – Ulcers >10mm with an irregular/oval shape and grey base. They last from 2 weeks to 3 months and importantly scar on healing.
> - *Herpetiform type* – Ulcers are very small (0.5–3mm) with a round shape and may coalesce. They have a yellowish base with erythema at the border, lasting for 1–2 weeks and heal with no scarring.

Appropriate investigations include bloods to include a full blood count, haematinics and zinc assay. Other blood tests might include testing for coeliac antibodies.

MANAGEMENT

Much of the management is centred around exclusion of an underlying abnormality (such as Crohn's disease or iron deficiency anaemia). If such causes are found, they should be treated accordingly.

Options for treatment include:

- Symptomatic relief with mouthwashes such as Difflam™, steroid-based mouthwashes (e.g Prednesol™ (soluble prednisolone 5mg tablet) or Betnesol™ (soluble betamethasone 0.5mg tablet), dissolved in 10ml of water and rinsed up to QDS when ulcers are present and OD when ulcer free) or steroid inhalers if they are isolated ulcers.
- For herpetiform ulceration tetracycline mouthwashes are often used.
- Any ulceration which fails to settle with these 'simpler' remedies might be more appropriately managed by the oral medicine team who are able to utilise immunosuppressive medications such as azathioprine, cyclosporin, colchicine and thalidomide.

LICHEN PLANUS/LICHENOID REACTION

This is a common condition, which can affect both the skin and oral mucosa. Although there are several variants of this disease, classically the patient will present with a 'white patch' in the mouth (Fig 4.2). The lesion may be noticed on routine dental examination, noticed by the patient asymptomatically, or referred because of pain and discomfort. The aetiology remains unclear and treatment is essentially symptomatic rather than curative. Oral lesions tend to last longer than concurrent skin lesions.

ASSESSMENT

- Exclude other mucosal disease
- Biopsy is indicated to confirm the diagnosis and exclude any dysplastic change
- Superimposed candida infection can often complicate this diagnosis, so prior to biopsy, exclusion of candida and treatment needs to occur (as candida hyphae seen histologically prevent detection of underlying dysplasia)
- It is prudent to remember that lichen planus in certain forms (atrophic and erosive and lichen planus, Fig 4.2) and anatomical areas are prone to dysplastic change and can be considered pre-malignant

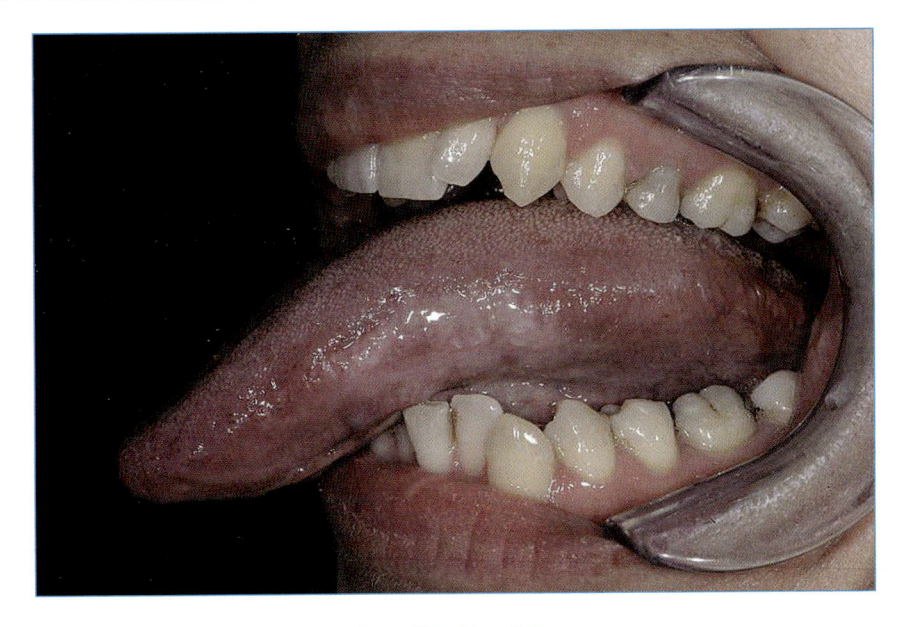

Fig 4.2. Lichen planus of the left lateral border of the tongue

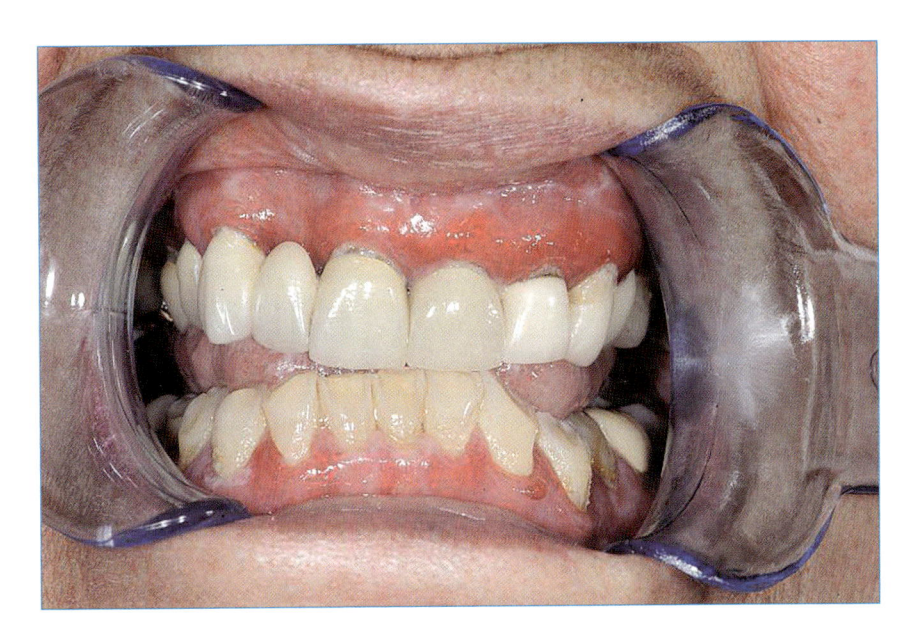

Fig 4.3. Erosive lichen planus with evidence of desquamative gingivitis (increased risk of dysplastic change)

An important differential for lichen planus is lichenoid reaction. This is commonly (but not always) unilateral and can be caused by the following:

- Drugs including gold therapy. Other medications include some antibiotics, NSAIDs, drugs used for treating hypertension, heart disease and high lipids.
- Restorative dental materials including amalgam-based restorations or toothpastes, particularly those are spearmint based. These may be identified by patch testing.
- Mechanical trauma
- Viral infection, in particular Hepatitis C

MANAGEMENT

There is no cure for lichen planus and patients should be counselled as such. Management is therefore supportive:

- Optimise oral hygiene
- Pain relief (e.g. Difflam™ mouthrinse)
- Topical (see page 126) and oral steroids
- Immunosuppressant medications may be required if severe

FIBROMA

Fibromas (fibroepithelial polyp), often referred by both GPs and GDPs, are soft tissue lesions of the oral mucosa or tongue (Fig 4.4), commonly the buccal or labial mucosa. They occur in response to local trauma, for example cheek biting, and appear as sessile or pedunculated lesions that are firm, smooth and painless on examination. Management involves simple excisional biopsy and histological analysis.

MUCOCELES

This is one of the commonest forms of minor salivary gland cyst, often known as a mucous extravasation cyst. There may be a history of precipitating trauma and patients will report a swelling which recurs on a cyclical basis and then settles after bursting spontaneously. On examination there will be a mobile, non-tender, fluctuant, round lesion palpable beneath the mucosa, and if superficial they may have a bluish/translucent colour. They commonly occur in the lip but also the buccal or labial mucosa.

They are treated with simple surgical excision under local anaesthetic, with excision of the cyst and affected underlying gland. Technically there is a risk of recurrence with trauma to adjacent minor salivary glands. Permanent numbness over the surgical site is a significant risk and patients should be warned of this pre-operatively.

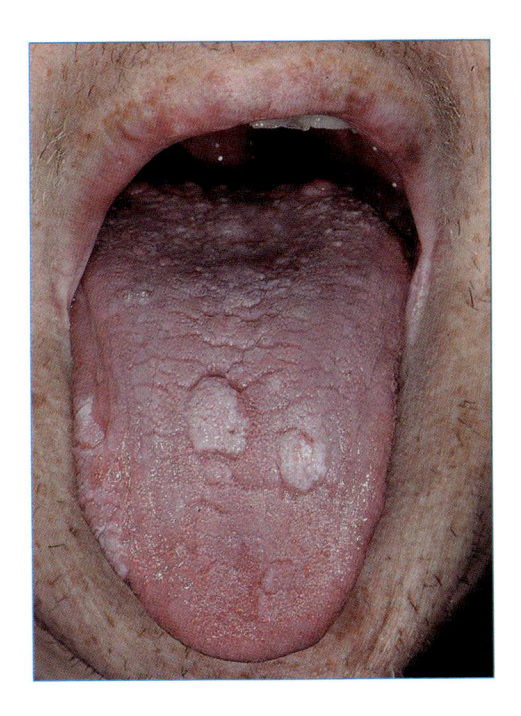

Fig 4.4. Multiple fibromas of the dorsum of the tongue (with right lateral border lichen planus)

ORAL CANDIDIASIS

While it is usually not a discrete soft tissue lesion within the mouth; oral candidiasis is included as it is a common presentation, that can have several forms and with differing symptoms. Acute (pseudomembranous) oral candidiasis can present with a classic creamy/white coating of the tongue or mucosa, with the patient complaining of an altered/bad taste. Wiping away of the white slough may reveal an inflamed erythematous underlying mucosa. However, chronic hyperplastic candidiasis can present as a white or white and red patch, often difficult to exclude from other conditions, such as lichen planus. Candida is also implicated in other chronic conditions such as angular chelitis, median rhomboid glossitis and denture-related stomatitis.

MANAGEMENT

Consider an underlying cause, such as immunocompromise, poorly controlled diabetes, medications (such as steroids or antibiotics) or patients with dentures; and manage/treat these accordingly.

It is best practice to confirm the diagnosis of oral candidiasis before starting antifungal medication, usually with a saliva 'spit' sample, to show high levels of candida. Suspicious white/red patches will usually need to be biopsied to confirm candida or other pathology. However, if clinical suspicion is high then oral antifungals can be started without a definitive diagnosis.

- 1st line treatment is usually oral Nystatin 2-4ml (100,000 units/ml) QDS for 5–7 days. Alternatively consider a topical azole, such as Miconazole (Daktarin®) 5-10mls QDS for 5–7 days (used for denture-related stomatitis).
- If a severe infection, resistant to Nystatin, or in an immunocompromised patient, consider a systemic azole such as Fluconazole 50mg PO OD for 7–14 days.

NON-HEALING ULCER

Any non-healing ulcer that is present for 3 weeks or more, where no other clinical cause has been identified, is a suspected malignancy until proven otherwise. The patient should be referred on an urgent basis with the referral letter specifying the clinical concern. This is typically undertaken via a 'two week wait' cancer referral pathway.

An important and common differential diagnosis includes traumatic ulceration (such as that caused by a denture or tooth), where the ulcer will be well demarcated with an obvious margin. However, if there is no obvious traumatic component (either from a denture or a tooth), a biopsy should be undertaken to exclude a dysplastic process.

For features suggestive of malignancy and its management, see 'Suspected oral malignancy' page 131.

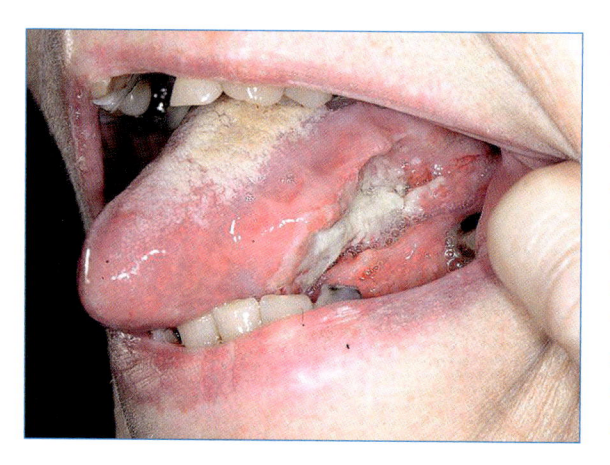

Fig 4.5. A large non-healing ulcer of the left lateral border of the tongue. The edges are clearly demarcated border, with rolled borders, a sloughy base with fibrin deposition. These findings are suggestive of a malignancy, commonly a squamous cell carcinoma.

SUSPECTED ORAL MALIGNANCY

Many patients with a suspected oral malignancy will be referred in by their GP or GDP and will be seen on a designated fast track clinic. The commonest primary oral malignancy is a squamous cell carcinoma.

As a general rule, any patient with a new or changing white/red patch or non-healing ulcer in the oral cavity will be seen on such a clinic within two weeks of the referral being made. They will also be referred and seen in a similar manner if there is new-onset regional lymphadenopathy with no obvious cause in the neck.

> Features that should raise the index of suspicion regarding a possible intraoral malignant lesion include:
> - Any non-healing ulcer that is present for 3 weeks or more, where no other clinical cause has been identified
> - Ulceration with a raised/indurated border
> - Painless red or white speckled patches in the mouth
> - Change in previously stable areas of lichen planus
> - Paraesthesia of the area or associated tongue pain or earache +/- dysphagia
> - Mobility of any adjacent teeth
> - Non healing tooth socket
> - Associated regional lymphadenopathy
> - Heavy tobacco/alcohol intake, especially in combination

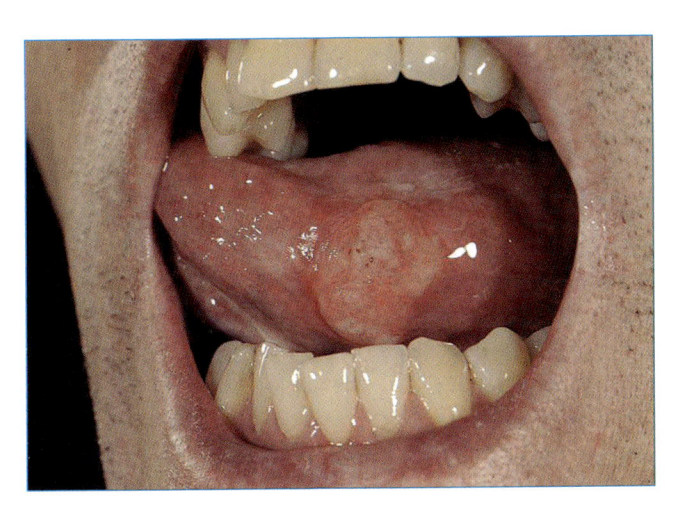

Fig 4.6. A suspicious lesion of the left lateral border of the tongue, exhibiting several of the signs discussed in the box above

ASSESSMENT

Your assessment should seek to identify risk factors and features suggestive of an oral malignancy (see box above), and then act to investigate these further.

Take a thorough history, with emphasis on a comprehensive medical history. For example, are they on medication that may have caused an ulcer (such as nicorandil), or will they be fit enough to undergo further investigations without optimisation? An accurate smoking and alcohol history requires documentation alongside any positive family history of oral cancer. Perform a detailed examination of the lesion in question, the entire oral cavity and regional neck lymph nodes.

INVESTIGATION

The findings from your clinical examination should lead to directed investigations. At this stage patients should be counselled about the possibility of 'cancer' as well as alternative diagnoses. Any ulcer or abnormal soft tissue requires an urgent biopsy. An OPG can be performed to screen for gross bony involvement. Once a tissue diagnosis has been obtained (from biopsy) then a CT head, neck and chest is required to stage the tumour.

On some occasions, biopsy under LA is not appropriate so the patient will need to be booked for an examination under general anaesthetic (EUA) with biopsies as required (hence the importance of a comprehensive medical history on initial review).

MANAGEMENT

Once tumour stage and grade has been determined, the case will be discussed in the head and neck MDT meeting to determine further management.

TMJ PRESENTATIONS

For many juniors, TMJ pathology is difficult to understand and manage alone. Increasingly, this group of patients is managed by specialist surgeons. However, these are not available in every unit. The following section will provide a brief guide on the assessment and management of such patients; to help you decide which patients can be managed locally, and which need to be referred on for more specialist input.

HISTORY

- What is the presenting complaint? This will often include pain, joint clicking/locking and reduced mouth opening.
- Take a thorough pain history and use a 10-point visual analogue scale to grade its severity.
- Is the pain myofascial in origin or in the distribution of a specific nerve (neuropathic)?
- Ask about the duration and what impact the symptoms have on activities of daily living, such as eating and speaking.
- Do they have restriction of mouth opening? Were these symptoms gradual or sudden onset?
- Have there been previous episodes of TMJ locking or dislocation?
- Is the patient aware of any bruxism or clenching?
- Are the symptoms associated with a predisposing event or trauma?
- What treatments have they tried? Which healthcare professionals have they seen previously?
- Take a full dental history, paying particular attention to previous orthodontic treatment or occlusal modification.
- Enquire about other systemic joint disorders.

EXAMINATION

- Mandatory documentation should include maximal incisal opening (MIO, measured with calipers or a ruler), protrusive and lateral excursions.
- Inspect and palpate the TMJ superficially and with your finger placed in the external auditory meatus.
- Palpate for masticatory muscle tenderness, hypertrophy (masseter and temporalis) and the presence of myofascial pain trigger points.
- Assess the patient's occlusion.

- Inspect for intraoral soft and hard tissue stigmata of bruxism (e.g. scalloping of the tongue, or evidence of hyper keratosis / ulceration of the cheeks, teeth wear facets).

INVESTIGATION

- An OPG is mandatory for the review of these patients as 1 in 10 will have some co-existing dental pathology that requires treatment (and may account for their symptoms). Inspect the condyles and comment on any obvious bony pathology (flattening/ bony spurs, absence). A degree of asymmetry between the two heads can be normal, so discuss this with your senior if in doubt. Also comment on the height of the joint space, which may be reduced/absent.
- CT and MRI are used to formally evaluate the joint and are used in planning prior to TMJ replacement.

DIAGNOSES

Having completed your assessment and initial investigations, you should have a list of diagnoses to confirm/exclude. In a patient presenting with pain, based on the elicited signs and symptoms, it is important to identify whether the pain is truly TMJ in origin, myofascial, neuropathic or atypical in nature (see 'Facial and oral pain' page 136).

Confusion continues to exist with the varying terminology used to describe TMJ disease. The term 'internal derangement' of the TMJ refers to an abnormal relationship of the TMJ disc to the joint itself. This results in disc displacement/slipping and the sound of clicking or locking of the TMJ as a result. The term TMJ (pain) dysfunction syndrome (TMJDS) is an all-encompassing term describing the condition of myofascial pain and TMJ tenderness with limitation to mouth opening and TMJ disc displacement (e.g. clicking/locking experienced by the patient). TMJDS is often used synonymously with the term Temporomandibular Disorder (TMD). The following are common specific TMJ pathologies to consider:

- TMJ dislocation/recurrent dislocation
- TMJ-related myofascial pain
- Anchored Disc Phenomenon (Acute Closed Lock)
- Degenerative Joint Disease, including ankylosis
- Condylar hyperplasia and idiopathic condylar resorption
- Missed mandibular condylar trauma with subsequent malocclusion/ deranged function

TREATMENT

Primary treatment is non-surgical with surgical intervention reserved for acute pathology or chronic refractory cases. Allow 6-8 weeks between interventions, and a longer period (at least 3 months) after surgical treatments.

Table 4.3: A brief overview of treatment options for TMJ-related myofascial pain and TMJ disorders.

TMJ-related myofascial pain

- Reassurance and patient education regarding the cause of the pain.
- Systemic/topical NSAID's.
- Superficial heat and cold therapy and massage.
- Use of a bite-raising appliance.
- If no response to above consider use of a low dose tricyclic antidepressant.
- Injection of Botox into areas of muscle spasm may also be beneficial.

TMJ disorders

- Apart from anchored disc phenomenon (see page 114), the majority of TMJ presentations should initially be treated as per myofascial pain (above), with reassurance, patient education, the use of regular NSAID's and a bite-raising appliance.
- Provide the patient with information leaflets detailing a series of TMJ exercises.
- Arthrocentesis is useful in those patients who have failed to respond to non-surgical treatment and is a useful diagnostic adjunct in cases where there is no history of trauma and the TMJ has previously not been accessed.
- If in doubt as to the benefit of arthrocentesis, consider the use of an injection of LA directly into joint space (e.g. Bupivicaine), which should achieve pain relief.
- Arthroscopy is used to evaluate the joint space in cases which subsequently represent after arthrocentesis with recurrence of symptoms, or in cases with a history of joint trauma. If required, it allows removal of any adhesions/spurs.
- Other surgical treatments include: meniscectomy/disc plication, condylectomy or total joint replacement.
- The use of steroid injections should be reserved for evaluation in specialist centres.

FACIAL AND ORAL PAIN

The complex anatomy of the face can make the diagnosis of facial and oral pain extremely difficult. A thorough pain history is vital, followed by relevant clinical examination. Initially dental pain should be excluded as a cause and following this, other diagnoses can be considered. Common presentations are discussed below, with additional diagnoses to consider listed in table 4.4.

TRIGEMINAL NEURALGIA

In trigeminal neuralgia, classically, the pain starts suddenly in the distribution of the trigeminal nerve, affecting the ophthalmic, maxillary and mandibular division (although the ophthalmic division is rarely involved). It is confined to these distributions and does not cross the midline. Pain is described as debilitating, triggered by touch/movement and may show a trigger pattern (which can be shaving in men or cold air on going outside, etc.). However, there is no sensory loss on formal examination and often, even after investigation, no apparent cause or pathology.

IMMEDIATE MANAGEMENT

In acute presentations to the ED, patients can be managed with local treatment and reviewed in the outpatient clinic. Immediate management options include infiltration with LA (using lidocaine with adrenaline) and if pain has resolved with this test administration, this can be topped up with a longer acting anaesthetic such as 5-10ml of Marcaine. Occasionally inpatient admission is required for an aggressive approach to pain control, including IV fluids if eating/drinking is compromised due to the pain.

IN THE CLINIC

Revisit the history and examinination. Imaging should include an OPG to exclude any dental pathology. A MRI is often requested to exclude a space-occupying lesion and identify whether there is any vascular anomaly in the region of the trigeminal nerve root ganglion that might merit a neurosurgical review with subsequent intervention. In younger patients, multiple sclerosis is a differential diagnosis until excluded with a report of a normal MRI scan.

LONG-TERM MANAGEMENT

Analgesia alone is sometimes sufficient to control the symptoms and some patients will undergo spontaneous remission. However, other methods of medical treatment are frequently required and include anti-convulsants (e.g.

carbamazepine) or cryotherapy to the nerve itself (which can be performed under local anaesthetic). Depending on whether a manageable cause has been identified, microvascular decompression may be performed by the neurosurgical team.

ATYPICAL FACIAL PAIN

Atypical facial pain is a diagnosis of exclusion. The classic patient is a middle-aged female presenting with severe pain, varying in character and not related to underlying anatomy (e.g. nerve distributions). There is often a psychiatric history and notably sleeping and eating are not disturbed with pain. After excluding an organic cause, anti-depressants can be trialled.

BURNING MOUTH SYNDROME (ORAL DYSAESTHESIA)

Burning mouth syndrome most commonly affects middle-aged females (sometimes with an underlying psychiatric history). Patients complain of a classic triad of symptoms: burning sensation to the oral mucosa, subjective xerostomia (dry mouth) and altered taste. Management is to exclude haematological, nutritional, or other organic causes for the pain (e.g. iron and Vit B12 levels, candidiasis). Tricyclic anti-depressants have been shown to be of benefit (e.g. Nortryptiline).

Table 4.4. Other diagnoses to consider with facial and oral pain

Diagnosis	Notes
TMJ-related myofascial pain	See 'TMJ presentations' page 133
Myofascial pain syndrome	Myofascial pain with 'trigger point' tenderness. Manage as per TMJ-related myofascial pain (see page 135).
Periodic migrainous headache	Periodic attacks of unilateral 'burning' pain (often in the distribution of the maxillary division of the trigeminal nerve) that last up to 60 minutes.
Glossopharyngeal neuralgia	Rare. Shooting pain on swallowing. Manage as per Trigeminal Neuralgia.
Temporal arteritis	Pain in temporal region (>50 years age group) with temporal tenderness and non-pulsatile superficial temporal artery. ESR is elevated but treat on suspicion alone, due to ocular complications, with IV steroids and temporal artery biopsy to confirm.
Space occupying lesion	Specific neurological signs may be evident on examination. Obtain further imaging (CT/MRI)
Ramsay Hunt syndrome / Bell's Palsy	Ear/jaw pain preceding facial palsy, due to inflammation of facial nerve (associated with herpes zoster in Ramsay Hunt syndrome, with associated vesicles of the external auditory canal).
Multiple sclerosis	Can present with trigeminal nerve symptoms. Often difficult to diagnose, requires MRI.

PRE-OPERATIVE ASSESSMENT CLINIC

Once a patient has been listed for an elective procedure, they usually attend a pre-operative assessment clinic. Here the patient's medical history can be reviewed to ensure they are fit for their surgical procedure, any pre-operative tests that have not been done can be arranged, the procedure can be discussed with the patient again and formal consent can be taken and the patients drug chart can be finalised before admission.

HISTORY AND EXAMINATION

In the elective setting, it is essential to:

- Confirm the patient's identity
- Establish their understanding of why they are to undergo surgery
- Discuss their expectations post-operatively
- Confirm the peri-operative and post-operative management plan

A general history and examination (see 'Admission clerking for emergency and elective patients' page 7) ensures that the patient is fit for surgery and that there are no medical contraindications to proceed. Patients may have significant comorbidities which will need to be managed appropriately during the peri-operative period. Often the patient's physician may need to be consulted for specific advice on peri-operative management (e.g. glycaemic control in diabetics, warfarin dosing and VTE prophylaxis).

A brief examination specific to the patient's maxillofacial problem and proposed treatment should also be undertaken. A senior colleague has most likely already assessed the patient but it is important to check that their findings have not changed significantly prior to the surgical procedure.

DRUG CHART

Patients on certain medication need special attention and should be discussed with your senior and/or the anaesthetist prior to surgery. Some medication may warrant discussion with other hospital physicians. For example:

- *Patients on long-term steroids* – the extra physiological stress of surgery can precipitate an Addisonian crisis. Higher maintenance doses may be required peri-operatively.
- *Diabetics* – See 'What to do with diabetics before surgery' page 95.
- *Epileptics* – Patients on regular anticonvulsants may require higher/

lower doses in the presence of other medications used peri-operatively. If the patient has a history of poorly controlled epilepsy, discuss the patient with the hospital's neurologist prior to surgery.
- *Patients on antiplatelets (e.g. Aspirin, Clopidogrel, Dipyridamole) and/or anticoagulation (warfarin, heparins) prophylaxis* - Although potentially increasing peri-operative bleeding risk, such medications are prescribed for both primary and secondary prophylaxis against life threatening conditions so should not be stopped peri-operatively without careful consideration (see 'What to do with patient's on warfarin pre-operatively' page 110). It may require discussion with the haematology or cardiology team.
- *Hyperthyroidism and neck surgery* - Patients with hyperthyroidism/ thyrotoxicosis undergoing neck surgery (either partial thyroidectomy surgery for their disease or simply coincidental neck surgery e.g. neck dissection) are at risk of developing a 'thyroid storm' through intraoperative manipulation of thyroid tissue. Therefore discuss this potential risk with your senior and/or anaesthetist to see if extra/ higher dose thyroid-suppressing medication (e.g. carbimazole) is indicated peri-operatively.

'HOSPITAL SUPERBUGS'

Patients with a history of MRSA infection/colonization (or other antibiotic resistant organisms), a recent inpatient hospital admission or those from other healthcare institutions (nursing homes etc.) are at higher risk of MRSA infection and transmission. All elective patients are now swabbed pre-operatively for MRSA. Consult your hospital's infection control policy to ensure appropriate preventative measures are taken (e.g. side-room isolation, chlorhexidine body scrub, mupirocin nasal ointment, contact precautions).

PRE-OPERATIVE INVESTIGATIONS

These should be general (relating to the patient's fitness for surgery) as well as specific to the procedure undertaken.

ECG

- Essential in anybody with known cardiovascular or respiratory disease or with cardiac risk factors.
- Usually performed routinely in those over 50 years old.
- This should be reviewed by somebody with experience in ECG pattern recognition.

BLOOD TESTS

Essential in those undergoing a lengthy general anaesthetic procedure (not always necessary in short procedures in young fit people):

- Full Blood Count – to ensure the patient is not anaemic, leukopaenic or suffering from systemic infection
- Biochemistry – to check renal function and electrolyte balance

If the procedure is long or there is a significant bleeding risk:

- Clotting screen (with INR if on warfarin)
- Group and Screen – This bottle often needs to be labelled by hand to help prevent administrative errors and ultimately mismatch in the event of blood transfusion (check your local protocol). If the procedure is associated with a high bleeding risk, an appropriate quantity of blood should be requested to be cross-matched and available on the morning of surgery. In cases where blood will definitely be required, a typical starting point would be to request two units of packed red cells pre-operatively. However, this will vary based on local protocol and procedure. If there is any doubt then liaise with the operating surgeon.

Other specific blood tests:

- Random blood glucose or fingerpick 'BM' (in diabetic patients)
- Liver function tests and amylase (in patients with a history of pancreatic or hepatobiliary disease)
- Bone profile tests (in patients with disorders of calcium metabolism or surgery affecting the parathyroid glands)
- Thyroid profile tests (in patients with thyroid disorders or surgery affecting the thyroid gland)

CHEST X-RAY

- Essential in anybody with cardiovascular or respiratory disease
- Often performed routinely in the elderly population

OTHER IMAGING

This is usually performed long-before admission for elective surgery and may include:

- CT/CT Angiography (e.g. prior to microvascular free-tissue transfer procedures)
- MRI/MR Angiography
- Lymphoscintigraphy (e.g. within 24 hours of sentinel node biopsy procedures)

- Ultrasound (or perhaps ultrasound-guided pre-operative skin marking of subcutaneous lesions/vasculature etc.)

OTHER SPECIFICS (FOR EXAMPLE...)
- Ensure that the patient's model and articulator are available prior to orthognathic surgery
- Ensure pre-operative imaging (OPG/plain films, CT, MRI etc.) is available for intraoperative viewing

CONSENT

See 'Consenting a patient for surgery' (page 142) for more information. Consent should be done in good time before taking the patient to theatre. In the elective setting, it is often done in the pre-assessment clinic as it allows the patient time to consider the risks and benefits of the procedure, giving them an opportunity to ask any questions they have before the day of the surgery. If you do not feel confident to be able to answer these questions, defer the consent-taking process to your senior.

WHERE TO PUT PATIENTS ON AN OPERATING LIST

In hospitals there are generally two types of operating lists: emergency and elective. A consultant will have their own day elective list, whereas the hospital emergency list is shared by all specialties and allocates patients based upon urgency categories (immediate, urgent, expedited, elective).

While it is unlikely to be your job to structure an elective operating list, it is not uncommon to be called by the operating theatre co-ordinator, especially with emergency operating lists, asking questions such as *'Which patient do you want to go first on today's list?'*.

The following tips give some advice for common scenarios and issues when structuring an inpatient list. It is easier to consider patients that should go first or last on a operating list, but clearly your clinical judgment will always be required. If in doubt consult your on-call senior.

FIRST ON OPERATING LIST	LAST ON OPERATING LIST
Children	MRSA positive patients
Diabetic patients	Minor operations (or first on list)
Patients with latex allergy	Operations under LA (or first on list)
Major operations	

CONSENTING A PATIENT FOR SURGERY

GUIDELINES ON CONSENT

These notes are guidance only. The complex legal nature of consent can produce very difficult situations, both for the doctor and the patient. If in doubt, consult your on-call senior.

CONSENTING FOR PROCEDURES

To consent for a procedure you must be suitably trained and qualified with sufficient knowledge of the treatment and risks involved. For junior clinicians this may pose limitations. Therefore, the caveat to this section is that upon starting your job you should discuss with your team which surgical procedures you and they are happy for you to consent for.

Consent is dependent upon an informed decision to proceed with an operation or procedure. A patient must have the capacity and be mentally competent to consent. They must understand the information you are telling them, retain it and weigh up the risks and benefits in order to make their decision. In some situations you may require a translator to aid understanding.

OBTAINING CONSENT

- Confirm the patient's identity, both verbally and by patient's identity bracelet.
- Explain the reason for the operation, the nature of the operation and if needed, how it will be carried out.
- Explain the risks and benefits of the operation.
- Explain any alternatives to the operation and the consequences of not having the operation.
- Ask if the patient has any questions.

When filling out any consent form:

- Write the procedure in clear legible handwriting.
- Specify side and site (where possible mark the operative site).
- Do not use abbreviations.
- Detail the benefits and risks of the procedure, as listed and discussed with the patient.

Individual risks and benefits for common operations are listed at the end of this section.

TRICKY SITUATIONS WITH CONSENT

UNCONSCIOUS ADULT UNABLE TO CONSENT

This is mostly encountered in emergency situations. In this circumstance the patient is obviously unable to provide valid consent or refusal to consent to the operation.

The decision to proceed is made by the patient's lead physician. This is applicable if the operation:

- Is life-saving
- Is to prevent a serious deterioration in the patient's health

ADULT WITHOUT CAPACITY TO CONSENT

No adult can consent on behalf of another for any procedure or operation. The difficulty with this group of patients is when capacity is questioned or in doubt. Such circumstances include elderly patients with a history of dementia, or patients with a mental health disorder.

- Capacity is best assessed by the person taking the consent
- If in question, a formal capacity assessment should be undertaken, often by more than one member of the team (i.e. doctor and nurse)
- It is not the job of the psychiatric team to attend the ward and assess capacity

Advance directives or living wills must be respected as the patient's wishes prior to their current state, unless you have reason to believe that the patient has changed their mind. Similarly the known wishes of a patient, either from a family member or regular medical practitioner, can be taken into account when deciding on a course of treatment.

CHILDREN

A child over the age of 16 is considered an adult and can consent for an operation. Children under the age of 16 must be assessed on an individual basis to determine if they have the understanding and ability to consent for a procedure. This is colloquially termed 'Gillick competence' (after a high-profile UK court case).

A child not deemed to have the competence to consent must have consent given by a person deemed to have 'parental responsibility'.

If the parents refuse treatment that is in the child's best interests, you must act to 'do good' and seek medico-legal advice, possibly culminating in legal action.

BENEFITS AND RISKS OF SPECIFIC SURGICAL PROCEDURES

The following section details information typically included on the consent form for the commonest OMFS procedures conducted in the emergency and elective setting. These lists are not exhaustive and serve as a guide only. Benefits and risks of surgery should be discussed using language and terms that the patient can fully understand.

OPEN REDUCTION AND INTERNAL FIXATION OF MANDIBLE FRACTURE(S)

BENEFITS OF THE OPERATION

- Aid healing
- Restore function (chewing)

POSSIBLE RISKS OF THE OPERATION

- Pain, swelling, bleeding, bruising, infection (early/late)
- Non-union/mal-union
- Paraesthesia of inferior alveolar or mental nerve (permanent vs. temporary)
- Injury to marginal mandibular branch of facial nerve (if using a transbuccal/extraoral approach)
- Extraction of teeth (requiring extraction if impairing reduction of fracture)
- Damage to adjacent teeth/restorations
- Post-operative malocclusion
- Loss of vitality of teeth adjacent to fracture line
- Scar (if transbuccal/extraoral approach)
- Temporomandibular joint dysfunction syndrome
- Possibility of requirement for plate removal if late infection/smoker
- Need for revision procedures

INCISION AND DRAINAGE OF OROFACIAL/NECK-SPACE COLLECTION

BENEFITS OF THE OPERATION
- Treat infection and prevent deterioration
- Restore function

POSSIBLE RISKS OF THE OPERATION
- Bleeding, infection, scar, swelling, haematoma, pain.
- Weakness of the lower lip (through damage of the marginal mandibular branch of the facial nerve)
- Intraoral drainage of infections may damage the inferior alveolar/dental nerve (leading to lip and tooth numbness) or the lingual nerve (leading to numbness of the anterior tongue)
- Extraction of teeth
- Damage to teeth or restorations
- Placement of an intra or extraoral drain
- Repeat drainage at a later date

MANIPULATION UNDER ANAESTHESIA OF NASAL BONE FRACTURE(S)

BENEFITS OF THE OPERATION
- Restore function
- Restore facial profile

POSSIBLE RISKS OF THE OPERATION
- Bleeding, infection, pain, swelling, haematoma (including septal haematoma)
- Residual deformity
- Nasal obstruction
- Need for revision procedure (septoplasty/septorhinoplasty)
- Need for nasal packs post-operatively

GILLIES LIFT (REDUCTION OF ZYGOMATIC ARCH FRACTURE)

BENEFITS OF THE OPERATION
- Restoration of facial profile
- Restore function
- Aid bone healing

POSSIBLE RISKS OF THE OPERATION
- Pain, swelling, bleeding, bruising
- Paraesthesia of infraorbital nerve (permanent or temporary)
- Temporal scar
- Possibly an intraoral access wound
- Residual asymmetry
- Diplopia
- Risk of retrobulbar haemorrhage

OPEN REDUCTION AND INTERNAL FIXATION OF ZYGOMATIC FRACTURE

BENEFITS OF THE OPERATION
- Restoration of facial profile
- Restore function
- Aid bone healing

POSSIBLE RISKS OF THE OPERATION
- Pain, swelling, bleeding, bruising
- Paraesthesia of infraorbital nerve (permanent or temporary)
- Need for upper eyelid incision (eyebrow/upper blepharoplasty type)
- Need for lower eyelid incision (cutaneous/transconjunctival for example)
- Temporal scar
- Possibly an intraoral access wound
- Residual asymmetry
- Diplopia
- Risk of retrobulbar haemorrhage

OPEN REDUCTION AND INTERNAL FIXATION ORBITAL FLOOR FRACTURE

BENEFITS OF THE OPERATION

- Restoration of function
- Improved aesthetics
- Promote bone healing

POSSIBLE RISKS OF THE OPERATION

- Pain, swelling, bleeding, bruising
- Risk of infection (early/late based on reconstructive material used)
- Paraesthesia of infraorbital nerve (permanent vs. temporary)
- Scar dependent upon access used
- Ectropion
- Entropion
- Diplopia (permanent vs. temporary)
- Loss of visual acuity secondary to a retrobulbar haemorrhage
- Late enophthalmos
- Epiphora/duct injury

BIMAXILLARY OSTEOTOMY

BENEFITS OF THE OPERATION

- Improved facial profile, function and occlusion
- Completion of orthognathic treatment plan

POSSIBLE RISKS OF THE OPERATION

- Pain, swelling, bleeding, bruising
- Risk of infection (early vs. late)
- Paraesthesia of inferior alveolar and lingual nerve (permanent vs. temporary) during the mandibular sagittal split osteotomy
- Infraorbital nerve paraesthesia (permanent vs. temporary) during the maxillary osteotomy
- Persistent malocclusion
- IMF post-operatively
- Continued use of elastics
- Change in facial profile/lip and nasal tip
- Use of intraoperative airway access such as submental intubations
- Removal of plates. Relapse

DENTAL EXTRACTION(S)

BENEFITS OF THE OPERATION
- Relief from pain
- Prevent spreading infection, decay in other teeth, pericoronitis (in impacted 3rd molars)
- For purposes of orthodontic treatment

POSSIBLE RISKS OF THE OPERATION
- Pain, bleeding, swelling, infection, bruising
- Dry socket
- Damage to adjacent teeth
- Requirement for a surgical procedure with bone removal, incision to mucosa and placement of mucosal stitches

RISKS SPECIFIC TO UPPER MOLARS/ 3RD MOLARS
- Fracture of maxillary tuberosity
- Oro-antral communication with need for further operative intervention

RISKS SPECIFIC TO LOWER MOLARS/3RD MOLARS
- Inferior alveolar nerve damage causing temporary or permanent pain, tingling or loss of sensation to the gums, teeth, lips and skin of chin.
- TMJ pain and risk of dislocation
- Fractured mandible

TRACHEOSTOMY

BENEFITS OF THE OPERATION
- Secure airway during the management of oral malignancy or complex facial trauma
- To aid long term respiratory support

POSSIBLE RISKS OF THE OPERATION
- Bleeding (early vs late)
- Infection
- Scar
- Pneumothorax/pneumomediastinum
- Subcutaneous emphysema
- Recurrent laryngeal nerve injury (hoarse voice)
- Oesophageal injury/tracheoesophageal fistula
- Inability to speak (unless fenestrated tube used)
- Airway obstruction
- Pneumonia
- Damage to trachea/tracheomalacia
- Tracheal stenosis
- Displacement of tube/accidental decanulation
- Failed healing

NECK DISSECTION

BENEFITS OF THE OPERATION
- To remove potentially malignant neck lymph nodes
- To minimise neck recurrence

POSSIBLE RISKS OF THE OPERATION
- Pain and swelling
- Bleeding, including damage to internal jugular vein and carotid vessels
- Scar
- Damage to recurrent laryngeal nerves, marginal mandibular nerves, accessory nerves, leading to change in voice, impaired swallowing, facial weakness and shoulder stiffness
- Chyle leak

PAROTIDECTOMY

BENEFITS OF THE OPERATION
- Removal of lump
- Confirmation of diagnosis

POSSIBLE RISKS OF THE OPERATION
- Pain, swelling, bleeding
- Recurrence of cancer or lump
- Facial weakness (temporary or permanent nerve injury)
- Frey's Syndrome (gustatory sweating)
- Salivary fistula
- Facial scar
- Change in soft tissue fullness in the region
- Further treatment dependent on final diagnosis

POST-OPERATIVE REVIEW CLINIC

Most patients who have undergone emergency and elective procedures will require a post-operative review. This is to ensure the patient is recovering well, appropriate healing is taking place and to identify those who require further intervention.

Common post-operative conditions seen on such clinics include the following:
- Mandible fractures
- Dento-alveolar fractures
- Midfacial fractures
- Orofacial and neck space infections
- Orthognathic osteotomies
- TMJ procedures
- Significant soft tissue injuries

MANDIBLE FRACTURES

These patients are often followed up to reinforce advice provided upon discharge. This will include the importance of a soft diet, avoidance of contact sports and avoiding smoking.

ASSESS AND DOCUMENT THE FOLLOWING:
- The patient's function and occlusion
- The presence of any altered sensation in the distribution of the inferior alveolar nerve
- Post-operative radiographic results for films taken on discharge
- If there is any clinical suspicion of a less than adequate reduction, if radiographs were not taken upon discharge, the first clinical attendance should prompt them
- Extraoral sutures have been removed and assess for any marginal mandibular nerve dysfunction if a transbuccal approach was utilised during operative fixation
- Intra and/or extraoral wound healing

FURTHER REVIEW

Occasionally, these patients might need additional support with the use of elastics applied to arch bars or Leonard buttons or IMF screws if these are still in-situ. Often these patients might also have an undisplaced condylar fracture and will continue to require a weekly review in order to ascertain the adequacy of IMF management.

If there is any suggestion of intraoral breakdown occurring, further regular review is essential. Such patients need to be told to continue with meticulous oral toileting.

Provided the patient's recovery proceeds uneventfully, a further review at 4–6 weeks is often sufficient, when if all is well, they can be discharged after removal of arch bars/Leonard buttons/IMF screws.

DENTO-ALVEOLAR FRACTURES

Often these patients are reviewed one week after injury, at which time any removable splints that have been applied can be removed, cleaned and replaced if needed.

Bony union takes approximately 6 weeks, therefore the importance of good oral hygiene, soft diet, minimal smoking and avoidance of contact sports during this period needs to be reinforced.

After isolated dento-alveolar fractures, if under the care of a GDP, the patient can be discharged back to GDP care, or should otherwise be encouraged to find a suitable practitioner.

MIDFACIAL FRACTURES INCLUDING THOSE OF THE ZYGOMATIC ARCH AND COMPLEX, ORBITAL FLOOR AND COMPLEX FACIAL FRACTURES

Initial review should ensure any skin sutures/staples have been removed entirely.

ISOLATED MIDFACIAL FRACTURES AND THOSE OF THE ARCH AND ZYGOMATIC COMPLEX

- Initial review will often lead to discharge
- The main purpose of assessment is to ensure there is no residual malocclusion or facial asymmetry
- Paraesthesia if present, may be resolving as a result of surgical correction, but may remain permanent. It is important to document this if present, and counsel patients accordingly.

ORBITAL FLOOR REPAIR
- Document visual acuity and pupillary response
- Ensure there is a full range of eye movements and assess any diplopia if reported. If diplopia is reported to be improving with normal eye movements, they can be reassured.
- Any diplopia with restriction or abnormality of eye movement should be reviewed by the ophthalmologist, orthoptist, and discussed with the treating surgeon. Formal evaluation with a CT scan may well be indicated. A repeat HESS chart may also be useful to assess for objective change.

Complex orbital floor fractures with any evidence of residual dystopia or telecanthus should be reviewed once all the swelling has resolved as there may be a role for further surgical input.

Many of the commercial products used for orbital floor fractures are designed to be left in-situ, but there is an increasing number of case reports emerging of patients having problems with some of these either resorbing, moving and/or causing infection at the surgical site at a later stage. Therefore, counsel patients about this and document this advice in the discharge letter to the GP so they are aware of where they need to return to and when.

ORTHOGNATHIC OSTEOTOMY PATIENTS

This review often occurs within the first week of surgery. Make sure you are familiar with what the surgical plan was intended to be. If you are in any doubt liaise with the treating surgeon.

Some surgeons will place their patients into elastics immediately post-operatively, others will wait until the first formal clinical review in order to allow swelling to settle.

ASSESS AND DOCUMENT THE FOLLOWING:
- Any issues with function and paraesthesia
- In the case of mandibular surgical procedures, is there a palpable step along the lower border of the mandible?
- If a genioplasty was performed, is there a step anteriorly?
- The post-operative occlusal result compared against planned outcome on models

- The adequacy of oral hygiene. If it is less than adequate, reinforce this with the patient.

If this appointment shows no issues, then further reviews are usually with the orthodontist alone, until the patient is ready for removal of their appliances, when they will attend a designated orthognathic clinic.

SIGNIFICANT SOFT TISSUE INJURIES

In the initial phase, attendance maybe to ensure sutures are removed. This usually occurs between 5 and 7 days. Removal of sutures can also be done at the patient's GP practice or local walk in centre. However, even if the patient reports this has been undertaken, you must still examine for and document that all sutures have been completely removed.

Once sutures are removed and the wound is dry, patients can be encouraged to use silicone-based products such as Dermatix® or Kelo-Cote®. Patients need to be aware that scars/abrasions will mature for approximately one year, and in this time care needs to occur to ensure no further sun damage compromises would healing. Application of at least factor 30 cream to facial scars is advisable.

In the instance of dirty/contaminated wounds, for example dog bites, ensure there has been no further episode of swelling or erythema and advise them upon the long term sequelae regarding scars.

If there is a significant facial deformity evident, a review at 6–8 months may well be indicated. Review and revision of such scars can be performed by the OMFS team, but occasionally can take place in conjunction with the dermatology and plastic surgery teams.

OROFACIAL AND NECK SPACE INFECTIONS

These patients are reviewed in order to:
- Ensure soft tissue swelling is reducing
- Review any extra oral scars
- Ensure trismus is suitably managed to prevent it becoming more pronounced in the continual healing phase

Patients who required surgical drainage of orofacial and/or neck space infections as a result of dental infection may not be registered with a GDP. Advice regarding dental care needs to be reinforced so that they understand the nature and importance of prevention by attending for routine dental checkups.

PROCEDURES

VENEPUNCTURE, IV CANNULATION AND TAKING BLOOD CULTURES

VENEPUNCTURE USING THE BD VACUTAINER® TECHNIQUE

The BD Vacutainer® is a phlebotomy system commonly used in hospitals worldwide and is frequently hailed as a safer alternative to using a needle and syringe. Your hospital may use a similar vacuum bottle system. The procedure below is an example of how to perform venepuncture and therefore acts as a guide only. You should be familiar with your local protocols on venepuncture technique.

This procedure is used for undertaking blood tests only. If your patient will need cannulation anyway, blood can be taken through the cannula at its insertion, saving him/her from multiple needle insertions (see IV Cannulation below).

Venepuncture is a relatively non-traumatic procedure so it is perfectly acceptable to use the most obvious vein available, typically in the anterior cubital fossa. Ensure that there is no pulsatility to the chosen vessel to ensure that you do not cannulate the brachial artery by mistake.

1. Explain the procedure to the patient and gain verbal consent.
2. Using an alcoholic disinfecting skin wipe, gently wipe the chosen area.
3. Apply a (disposable) tourniquet to the arm, above the venepuncture site. Disposable rubber tourniquets are best tied with a half-knot or in a bow so easily removed afterwards.
4. Allow the alcohol on the skin to evaporate before inserting the needle with the bevel pointing upwards (away from the skin). Insert the needle into the vein at approximately 45 degrees to the skin surface. You can use a Vacutainer® needle directly attached to the holder, or a 'butterfly' alternative where the needle is attached to the Vacutainer® holder through a length of plastic tubing which can be useful for small veins and 'difficult-to-reach areas'. Both methods are acceptable.
5. As soon as you are in the vein, hold the Vacutainer® holder steady with your non-dominant hand. If using the 'butterfly' needle device, you may find it necessary to apply a piece of tape to the needle to keep it still whilst manipulating the Vacutainer® holder and bottles.

6. One by one, place the required Vacutainer® blood bottles into the holder, keeping the holder steady with the needle in the vein at all times.
7. Once you have filled all necessary bottles, loosen the tourniquet before removing the needle (this minimises the formation of a subcutaneous haematoma from the venepuncture site).
8. Apply cotton wool to the venepuncture site with pressure and secure with a suitable dressing tape.
9. Safely dispose of sharps.

IV CANNULATION

The BD Venflon™ is a cannula system commonly used in hospitals worldwide. Your hospital may use a similar cannulation system. The procedure below is an example of how to perform IV cannulation and therefore acts as a guide only. You should be familiar with your local protocols on cannulation technique.

The choice of cannula and cannulation site depends on the reason for cannulation. 'Small' cannulas (22G – Blue, 20G – Pink) can be used for simple maintenance IV fluids. The 22G provides insufficient flow rate for IV contrast studies and both types are inadequate for rapid fluid resuscitation. However, sometimes small cannulas need to be used if only small veins can be found. In which case, you may need to insert more than one cannula in order to provide sufficient quantities of intravenous fluids/medication. 'Medium' cannulas (18G – Green) are appropriate for both maintenance fluids and administration of larger boluses. 'Large' cannulas (16G – Grey, 14G – Orange) are generally used for administration of large fluid boluses and multiple medications through one peripheral line. These cannulas generally require larger veins. As a general rule it is best to use the largest cannula you can for a chosen vein.

When choosing the vein, again think first of why cannulation is necessary. If it is to provide potentially life-saving resuscitation, you should not have qualms over using a large cannula in a large vein (e.g. antecubital fossa or the cephalic vein in the forearm). If you are cannulating simply to administer routine drugs and fluids, smaller veins on the back of the hands (or feet) may be more appropriate. This saves larger veins from damage in case they are needed later for emergency cannulation.

1. Explain the procedure to the patient and gain verbal consent.
2. Using an alcoholic disinfecting skin wipe, gently wipe the chosen area.

ON-CALL IN ORAL AND MAXILLOFACIAL SURGERY

3. Apply a (disposable) tourniquet to the arm, above the cannulation site. Disposable rubber tourniquets are best tied with a half-knot or in a bow so easily removed afterwards.
4. Allow the alcohol on the skin to evaporate before inserting the needle with the bevel pointing upwards (away from the skin). Remove the cap from the cannula tip. Insert the needle with cannula sheath intact into the vein at approximately 45 degrees to the skin surface.
5. Once you have the needle tip in the vein, a flash-back of blood will be seen at the other end of the cannula hub. At this point, hold the needle component still (at the rear end of the cannula hub) and advance the cannula sheath further down the shaft of the needle (into the vein) to its entire length.
6. Maintain pressure over the subcutaneous cannula sheath tip (now in the vein) with your non-dominant thumb and remove the needle entirely from the cannula hub. Safely dispose of the needle or safely place it aside for disposal after the procedure.
7. With your dominant hand, screw on the cannula cap.
8. Flush the cannula through the 'flush' port with normal (0.9%) saline.
   a. If the patient complains of pain or you see swelling around the cannula site, stop flushing. The cannula is in the wrong place (not in the vein). In which case loosen the tourniquet before removing the cannula (this minimises the formation of a subcutaneous haematoma from the venepuncture site) and apply cotton wool to the venepuncture site with pressure and secure with a suitable dressing tape.
   b. If the cannula flushes without difficulty, swelling or pain, secure it in place with a purpose-made cannula dressing, or alternatively with dressing tape.
9. It is useful for nursing staff if you document the date of cannula insertion on the patient's chart/notes and on the cannula dressing itself as this will need replacement after typically 72 hours (check local protocol).

PHLEBOTOMY AT CANNULA INSERTION

This can be performed by connecting a BD Vacutainer® holder with cannula adapter into the rear of the cannula hub, before attaching the screw cap onto the rear of the cannula hub (i.e. between steps 6 and 7 above). This technique should not be performed after flushing or using the cannula as a diluted sample of blood will be obtained.

BLOOD CULTURES

Many hospitals have a 'blood culture pack' with specific instructions and guidelines on how to take blood culture samples. An example of blood culture bottles is illustrated in Fig 5.1. An example of the basic technique for taking blood cultures is as follows:

1. Open the blood culture pack.
2. Flip the plastic lids off the culture bottles.
3. Wipe both rubber culture bottle tops with alcoholic chlorhexidine wipes/sponge.
4. Prepare the patient's arm as for venepuncture (tourniquet, alcohol wipe at site).
5. Take blood sample with a 20ml syringe and needle, remove tourniquet and apply dressing/cotton wool to venepuncture site.
6. CAREFULLY remove the needle and replace with a fresh sterile one.
7. Inject 5-10ml of blood into the AEROBIC culture bottle first
8. Inject 5-10ml of blood into the ANAEROBIC culture bottle second. Take care to ensure that any air in the syringe does not enter the anaerobic bottle.
9. Carefully dispose of your sharps and send the samples to the lab, signed and labelled.

Other techniques for taking blood cultures are available, including an adapted BD Vacutainer® system. Always consult your local hospital protocols.

ON-CALL IN ORAL AND MAXILLOFACIAL SURGERY   159

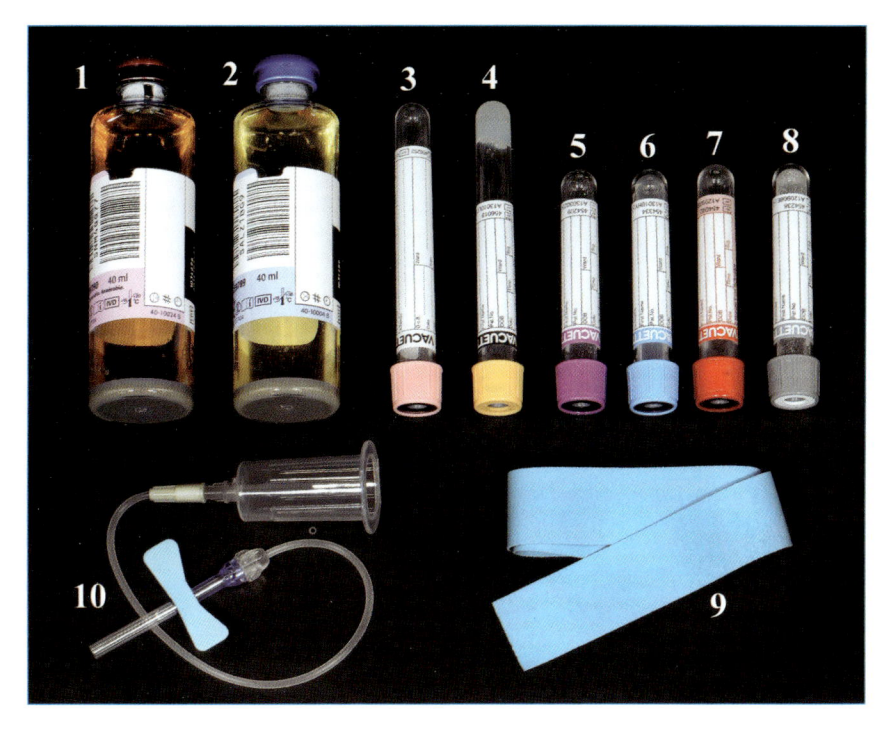

Fig 5.1. Assortment of blood culture bottles, BD Vacutainer® blood bottles and venepuncture equipment

1. Anaerobic blood culture bottle (purple top)
2. Aerobic blood culture bottle (blue top)
3. Cross match (pink top)
4. Biochemistry – SST™ II (yellow top)
5. FBC – EDTA (purple top)
6. Coagulation studies – Sodium Citrate (blue top)
7. Serum assays (red top)
8. Blood glucose, lactate – Fluoride Oxalate (grey top)
9. Disposable rubber tourniquet
10. Blue butterfly needle with Vacutainer® holder.

PROCEDURES

NERVE BLOCKS OF THE MOUTH AND FACE

Anaesthesia of the mouth and face is achieved either by infiltrating locally or blocking a specific nerve supplying a defined anatomical region. Due to the relatively thin maxillary alveolar bone, dental anaesthesia can be achieved by local infiltration in the area of the apex of the tooth/teeth. However, in the mandible this approach is unsuccessful and regional nerve blocks are required. We will discuss the technique to achieve regional anaesthesia, in the mouth and face, of each of the following nerves (Fig 1.9, 1.10 and 5.2):

- Inferior alveolar nerve (inferior dental nerve)
- Mental nerve
- Infraorbital nerve
- Supraorbital and supratrochlear nerves
- Ring block of the external ear

LOCAL ANAESTHETIC

LA is commonly used within the practice of OMFS, such as during facial laceration closure, or dental extractions, to achieve local or regional anaesthesia. As with any drug you administer, you must be aware of the mode of action, dosing and potential side effects and toxicity.

LAs are classified as either amides (lidocaine, bupivacaine, prilocaine) or esters (cocaine, procaine). They cause anaesthesia by reversible inhibition of cell membrane sodium channels and blocking the generation and propagation of action potentials.

Adrenaline is added to LA to cause localised vasoconstriction. This aids in haemostasis and also prolongs the duration of the LA by decreasing absorption. You should not use LA with adrenaline on areas of the face that have an end-arterial blood supply such as the ear or nose, as you risk ischaemic necrosis. The maximum doses for LA, described in Table 5.1, should be lowered in child and elderly patient populations.

Early symptoms of LA toxicity include perioral paraesthesia and light-headedness or dizziness. At higher doses, neurological symptoms may progress to drowsiness, confusion, seizures and even coma. Serious cardiovascular complications include bradycardia, hypotension and cardiac arrhythmias (ventricular fibrillation, asystole). The dose of LA in a cartridge is calculated using the percentage strength of the solution. As a rule: 1ml of a 1% solution equates to 10mg of the drug (1ml of a 2% solution is 20mg, etc).

Table 5.1. Maximum doses for commonly used anaesthetic agents

Anaesthetic agent	Maximum dose	Notes
Lidocaine	3 mg/kg	Used for short procedures (e.g. <60 minutes).
Lidocaine with adrenaline	7 mg/kg	
Articaine with adrenaline	7mg/kg	Useful for lower arch local infiltration to avoid ID block. Not used for ID block due to risk of neurotoxicity.
Prilocaine	6mg/kg	Safer in large doses.
Prilocaine with felypressin	8mg/kg	Useful when adrenaline is contraindicated (e.g. ischaemic heart disease). Avoided in pregnancy due to risk of inducing uterine contractions.
Bupivacaine	2 mg/kg	Used for longer procedures (e.g. >60 minutes).
Bupivacaine with adrenaline	2.5 mg/kg	

INFERIOR ALVEOLAR NERVE BLOCK

The inferior alveolar nerve has traditionally been referred to as the inferior dental nerve, leading to the colloquial use of the term 'ID block' when referring to this nerve block.

The ID block produces anaesthesia in the following regions (Fig 5.2):
- All ipsilateral teeth of one half of the mandible
- The ipsilateral gingivae and buccal/lingual mucosa of one half of the mandible
- The ipsilateral lip and skin of the cheek
- The ipsilateral half of the tongue

There are several ways to perform an ID block. Either with the mouth open or closed:
- *Direct standard ID block* – With the mouth open the needle is orientated above the premolar teeth and angled towards the mandibular foramen on the contralateral side.
- *Indirect standard ID block* – With the mouth open, as above, but the needle is initially placed over the ipsilateral teeth to aid placement then, once inserted into the mucosa, angled to lie over the contralateral premolars.

- *Gow-Gates technique* – With the mouth open, the needle is aimed at the condyle of the mandible.
- *Vazirani-Akinosi technique* – With the mouth closed, the needle is advanced parallel to the maxillary occlusal plane at the level of the maxillary mucogingival junction (useful in patients with trismus).

In this book, we describe the 'direct technique' which is reliable and relatively simple to perform. Patient positioning is important, but unlike in the dental outpatient environment, the patient may well be lying supine or even sat up in a chair. Therefore, a firm understanding of the anatomy of the block is vital to ensure appropriate delivery of the anaesthetic agent. Fig 5.4 and 5.5 show the plane where the anaesthetic should be delivered.

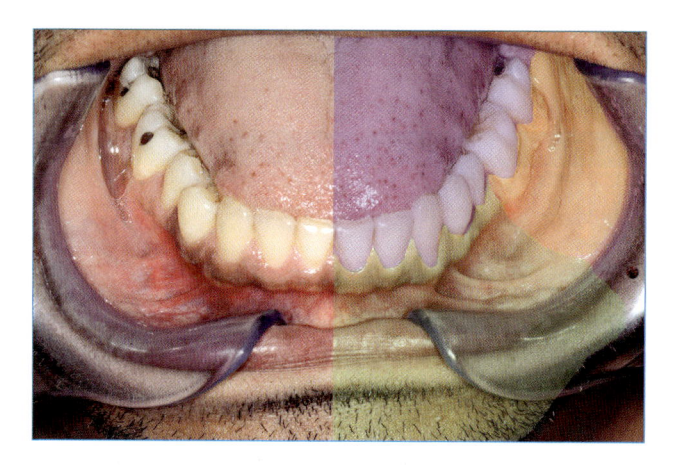

Fig 5.2. This picture demonstrates the regions of anaesthesia obtained with intraoral nerve blocks

- *Purple and Green region – ID block (through blocking the ID and lingual nerves)*
- *Green region – mental nerve block (including the chin and external lower lip)*
- *Yellow region – long buccal block*

1. Visualisation is often aided by tilting the patient's head slightly to the side of the block.
2. The external oblique ridge of the mandible can be palpated with the thumb.
3. The index finger can be used to gently support the posterior border of the ramus, which also helps provide the clinician with some idea of the width of the ramus.
4. The pterygomandibular raphe, where the superior constrictor meets the buccinators should be identified.
5. A long dental needle should be used. It should be oriented from the intended site of entry to the contralateral premolars (Fig 5.3).
6. The site of entry is described as the junction of the inferior and middle thirds of the inverted triangle ('V') formed by the pterygomandibular raphe and the external oblique ridge, or approximately 1cm above the occlusal plane (Fig 5.4 and 5.5).
7. The needle should be gently inserted. Generally the tip of the needle will contact the inner aspect of the ramus in this orientation at approximately 2.5cm, although this is highly variable from patient to patient. Once bone is gently felt, the needle can be withdrawn by approximately 1mm, gently aspirated to ensure the tip is not in a blood vessel, and 1-1.5ml of the anaesthetic gently injected.
8. In order to anaesthetise the buccal mucosa of the posterior teeth, it is often necessary to block the buccal nerve as well.
9. This block is achieved, often with the last 0.5 ml of the anaesthetic used for the ID block, by orientating the needle parallel to the teeth and entering the mucosa just distobuccal to the last molar (Fig 5.6).

POTENTIAL COMPLICATIONS OF AN ID BLOCK

- Trismus/jaw ache/stiffness – due to trauma to the medial pterygoid muscle
- Pain – subperiosteal haematoma due to trauma to ramus of mandible
- Dysphagia – involvement of the superior constrictor muscle
- Facial palsy – advancing too posterior and entering the parotid gland to anaesthetise the facial nerve

164 ON-CALL IN ORAL AND MAXILLOFACIAL SURGERY

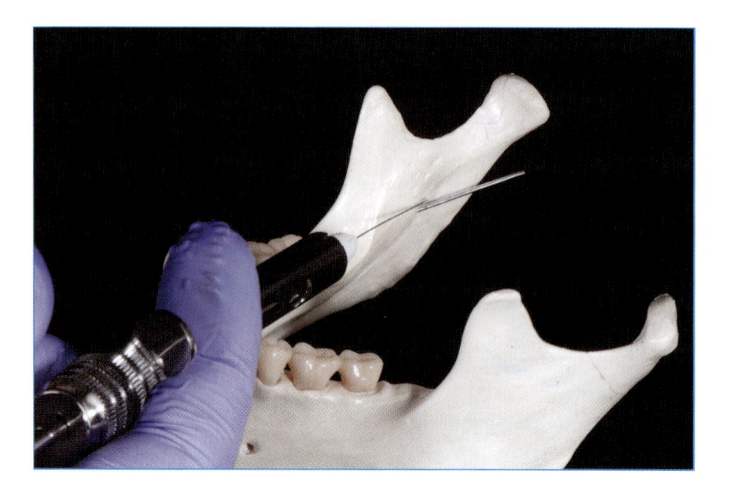

Fig 5.3. Mandible with pointer entering right mandibular foramen to simulate course of ID nerve. Demonstration of the position of the needle relative to teeth, bone, foramen and ID nerve.

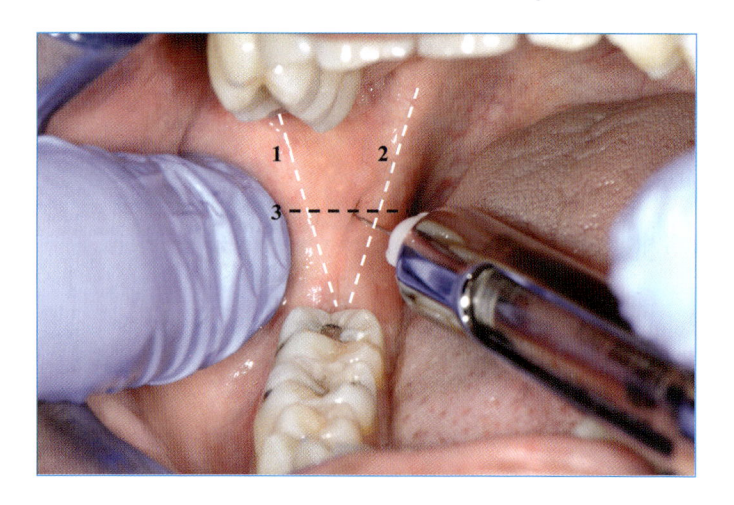

Fig 5.4. Performing an ID block. Anatomy highlighted to show 'V' landmark for needle placement.

1. External oblique ridge
2. Pterygomandibular raphe
3. Plane of transverse section described in Fig 5.5.

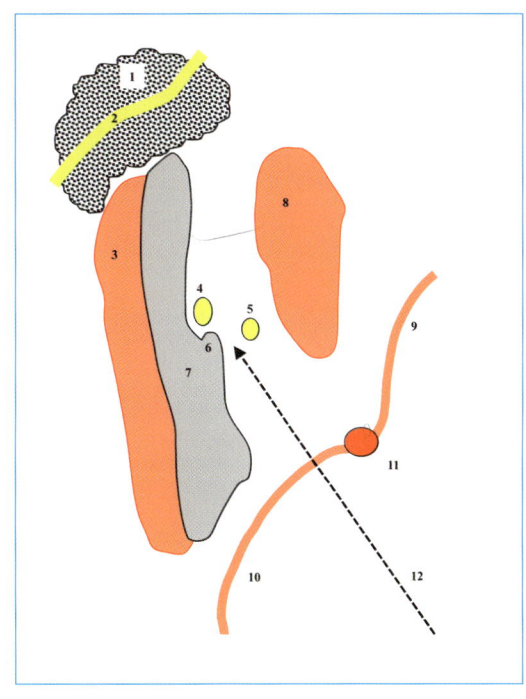

Fig 5.5. Transverse section at the level of line 3 on Fig 5.4. Demonstrating the relationship of the needle to the surrounding structures during an ID block.

1. Parotid gland
2. Facial nerve
3. Masseter
4. ID nerve
5. Lingual nerve
6. Lingula of mandible
7. Ramus of mandible
8. Medial pterygoid
9. Superior constrictor
10. Buccinator
11. Pterygomandibular raphe
12. Path of needle

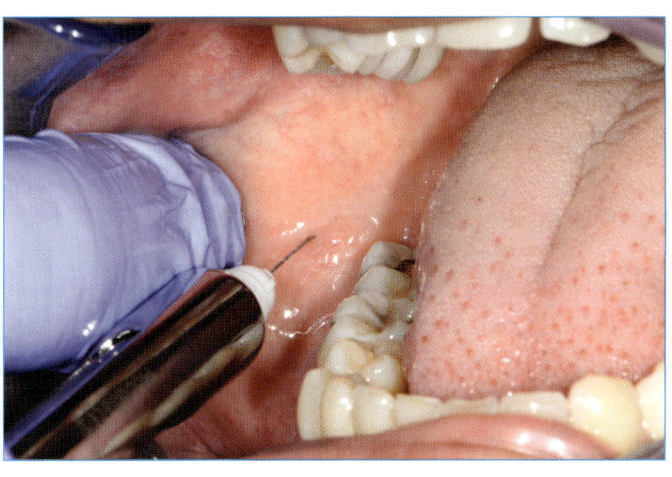

Fig 5.6. Performing a long buccal block

TOP TIPS

- Warn the patient to expect some discomfort. They are likely to experience a scratch at back of mouth with burning and pressure initially, then the lips may 'tingle' before going numb, along with the tongue and finally the teeth.
- Perform the ID block before long buccal to ensure that it is working properly.
- Inject very slowly to minimise pain.
- Sometimes for the most anterior teeth, local infiltration may also be required to achieve appropriate anaesthesia. This is due to contralateral supply from the opposite side of the arch, along with occasional sensory braches from the nerve to mylohyoid.

MENTAL NERVE BLOCK

This block is used to anaesthetise the ipsilateral lower lip, skin of the chin, mucosa and gingivae (Fig 5.2). It is simpler to deliver than the ID block and provides a more localised region of anaesthesia.

The mental foramen is located roughly halfway up the mandible between the apices of the two premolar teeth (4 and 5). It is sometimes possible to palpate the mental nerve as it emerges from the mental foramen. Its location can also be seen on an OPG.

1. The lower lip is pulled outwards to ensure the oral mucosa is under tension.
2. The needle is orientated in the direction of the long axis of the premolar teeth, angling slightly towards the bone.
3. The entry site for the needle is just above the anticipated site of the mental foramen in-between the premolar teeth

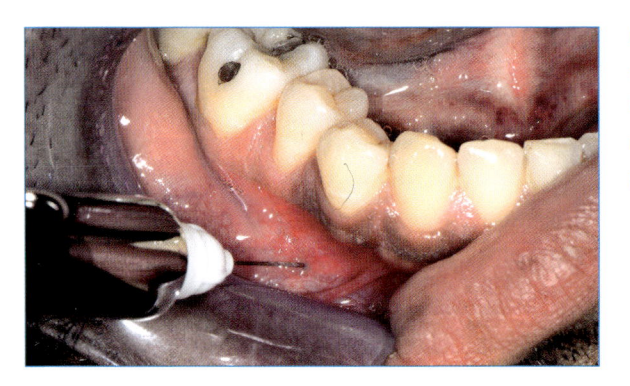

Fig 5.7. Performing a mental nerve block. Note position of needle between the premolars.

INFRAORBITAL NERVE BLOCK

The inferior orbital nerve is a terminal branch of the maxillary division of the trigeminal nerve. It emerges from the maxillary bone through the infraorbital foramen (Fig 1.6 no.6 and Fig 1.9). This is located approximately halfway along the length of the inferior orbital margin and approximately 1cm below it. It supplies sensation to the lower eyelid, the lateral aspect of the nose, the upper lip and anterior upper teeth.

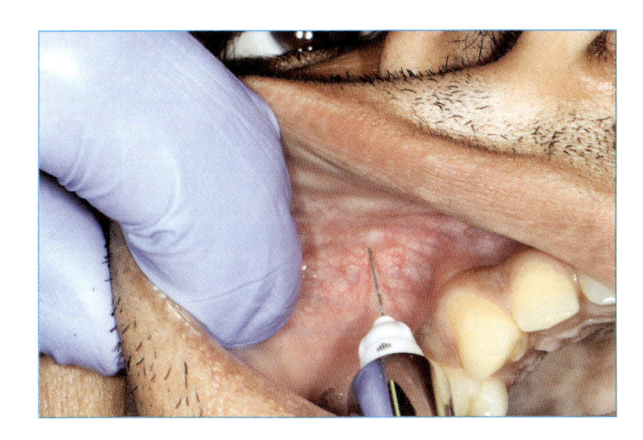

Fig 5.8. Performing an infraorbital nerve block

The block can be delivered via an extraoral or intraoral approach:
(a) The extraoral approach involves an injection of LA through the skin, in the mid pupillary line, 5mm inferior to the inferior orbital rim.
(b) The nerve can also be approached intraorally through the buccal sulcus of the upper jaw (Fig 5.8):

1. The index finger of the contralateral hand can be used palpate the position of the nerve during the procedure.
2. The buccal mucosa is again pulled taut.
3. The entry point of the needle should be between the canine and premolars.
4. A long (35mm) dental needle should be used and advanced until in the region of the infraorbital foramen, before gently aspirating and injecting the LA.

SUPRAORBITAL AND SUPRATROCHLEAR NERVE BLOCK

The supraorbital nerve supplies sensation to the upper eyelid, forehead and scalp (Fig 1.10). The supratrochlear nerve supplies sensation to a smaller area over the medial forehead and brow. Both nerves are branches of the frontal nerve, which in turn arises from the ophthalmic division of the trigeminal nerve. The supraorbital nerve emerges from the skull through the supraorbital foramen, although sometimes the foramen may be a notch in the edge of the superior orbital rim (Fig 5.9). The supratrochlear nerve emerges from the most supero-medial aspect of the orbital rim.

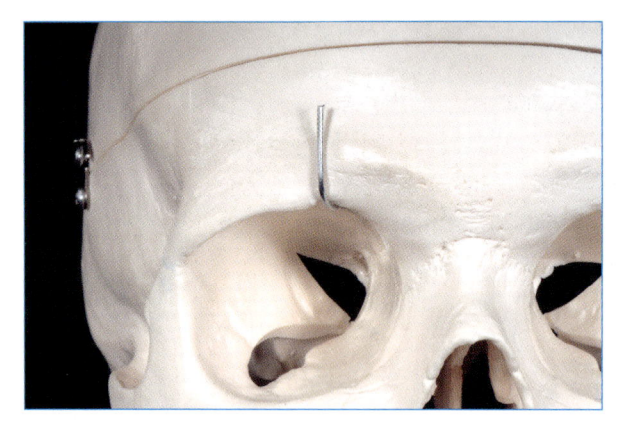

Fig 5.9. Skull with pointer simulating course of supraorbital nerve within supraorbital notch

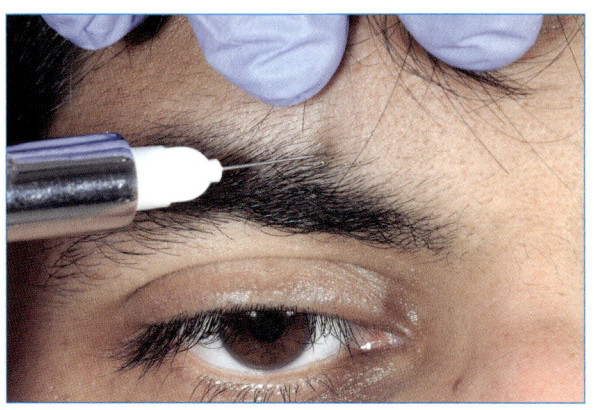

Fig 5.10. Performing a supraorbital nerve block

The supraorbital block is achieved by injecting LA in the region of the foramen/notch, thus anaesthetising the nerve as it emerges from the skull. The supraorbital foramen is located roughly at the centre of the superior orbital rim, and can be palpated as a notch in the rim itself.

Once located, using a sterile technique, the needle is introduced immediately superior to the notch. 1-2ml of LA can be administered after aspiration (Fig 5.10).

The supratrochlear nerve may already be anaesthetised by spread of LA from the supraorbital nerve injection. However, it can be further anaesthetised (immediately after injecting at the supraorbital foramen/notch), by advancing the needle medially along the supraorbital rim (approximately 1cm) and depositing a small amount (1ml) of LA there as well.

RING BLOCK OF THE EXTERNAL EAR

To anesthetise the external ear, a ring lock technique is used. This involves injecting LA (without adrenaline) around the base of the ear, in a 'ring' fashion, in order to anesthetise all nerves entering the ear.

The skin is prepped as for all injections. Two entry points are used, directly superior and inferior to the ear. LA is injected anterior and posterior to the ear form each entry point, to achieve the ring block (Fig 5.11).

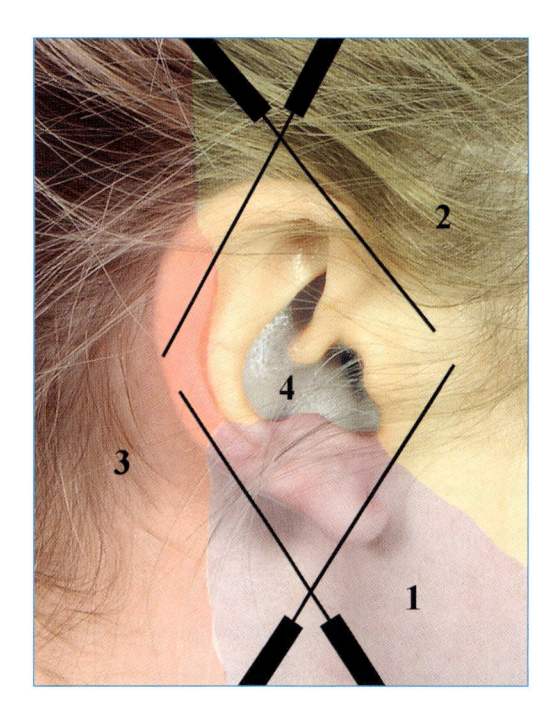

Fig 5.11. Ring block of the ear. Nerve supply to the external ear and needle injection sites shown in black lines.

1. Great auricular nerve
2. Auriculotemporal nerve
3. Lesser occipital nerve
4. Auricular branch of the vagus nerve

TOOTH SPLINTING

Tooth splinting is a method to stabilise a mobile tooth using support from neighbouring teeth. In the OMFS on-call setting, it is typically required after a traumatic injury to the tooth (see 'Dental Trauma' page 72). The aim is to reduce the tooth back into its original position and stabilise it to give the best chance of maintaining vitality and also alleviate pain. There are numerous methods and techniques and the following represents a guide only.

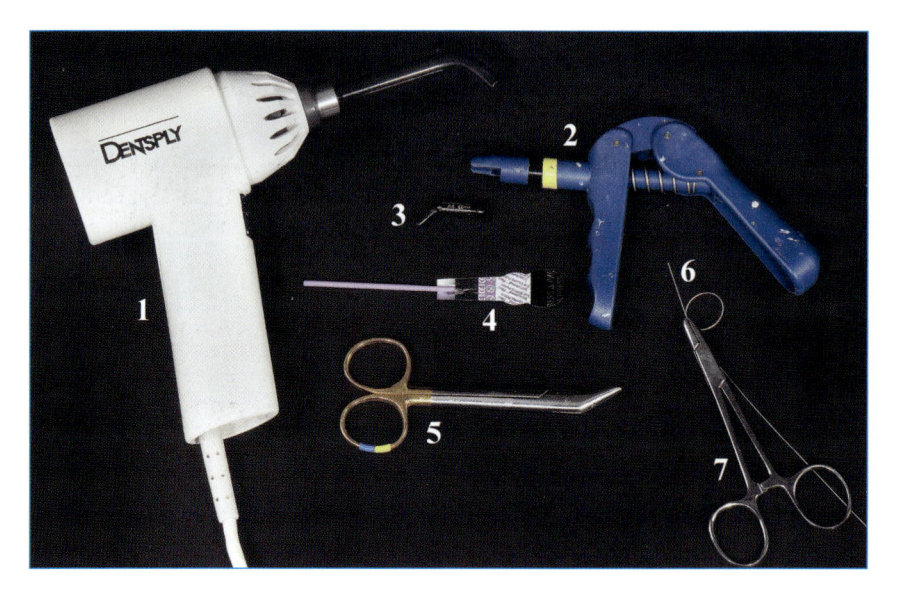

Fig 5.12. Dental instruments used when splinting a tooth with a wire-splint

1. *Light-cure gun*
2. *Composite gun*
3. *Composite ampule*
4. *All-in-one 'lollipop' etch, prime and bond system*
5. *Wire cutters*
6. *Orthodontic wire*
7. *Forceps*

ON-CALL IN ORAL AND MAXILLOFACIAL SURGERY 171

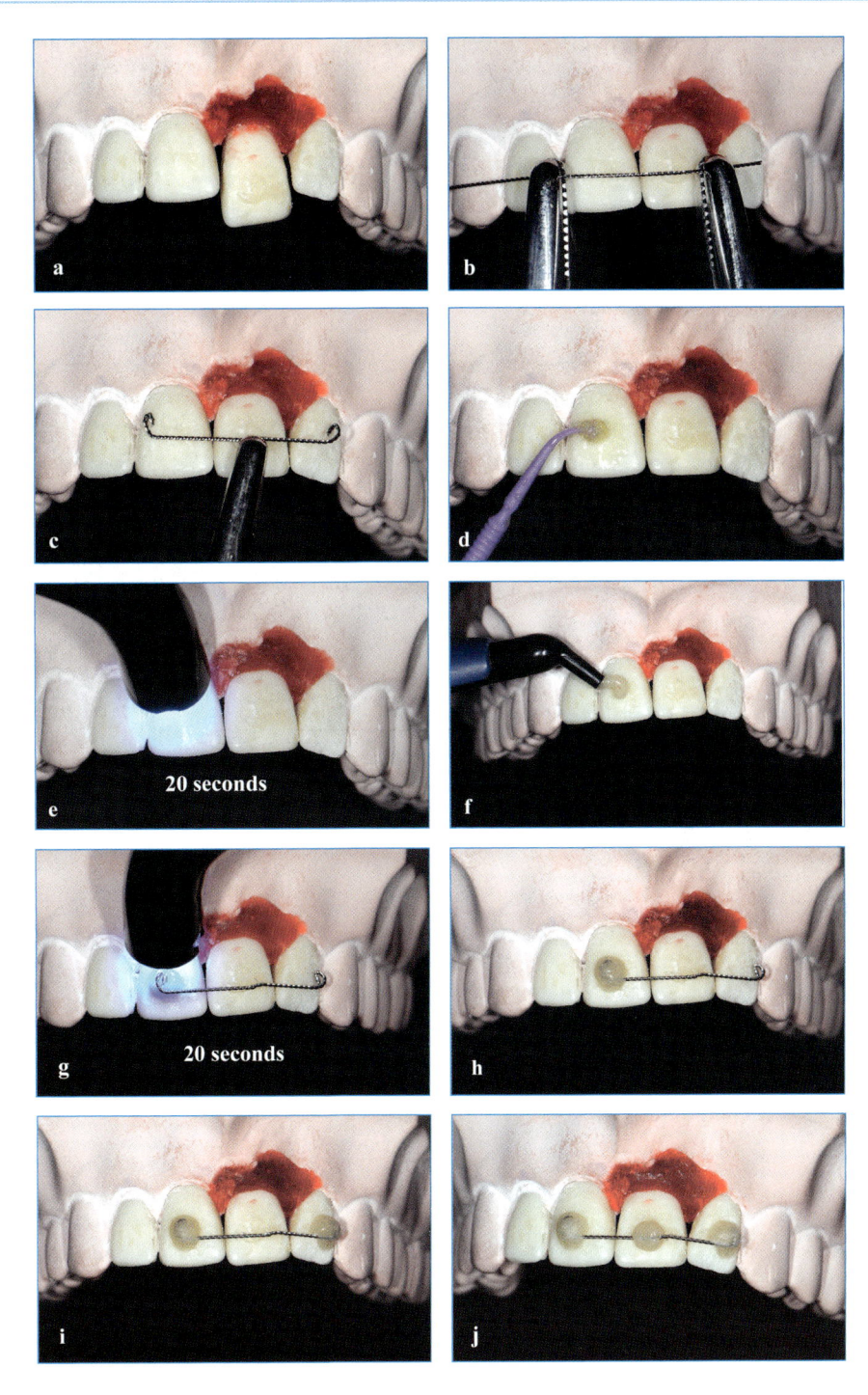

Fig 5.13. Tooth splinting procedure

PROCEDURES

FIG 5.13. TOOTH SPLINTING PROCEDURE

a) An upper left central incisor that has suffered dental trauma. The tooth is extruded and laterally luxated. Initially LA should be administered (either buccal infiltration or a regional block). The tooth should be reduced to its normal position using finger pressure, or it should be replacement in the socket if avulsed. Care should be taken to avoid touching the root surface.

b) A length of orthodontic wire is measured to the appropriate length - typically across 3-5 teeth: the avulsed tooth and 1-2 teeth either side.

c) The wire is cut and the ends are curled over to prevent soft tissue trauma. A dental (cotton wool) roll can be placed in the buccal sulcus to aid moisture control.

d) Either an 'all-in-one' etch and bond system can be used, or the tooth surface is etched and bonded in separate steps. This is applied to a dry tooth surface.

e) This is light-cured for 20 seconds.

f) A small amount of composite is applied over the etched and bonded area on the tooth/teeth on one side of the traumatised tooth.

g) The pre-cut orthodontic wire is then pushed into this until completely submerged. This is then light-cured for 20 seconds.

h) Further composite can be placed over the wire, and light-cured, to firmly secure the wire in place

i) The same process is repeated for all teeth lateral to the traumatised tooth.

j) Lastly, the traumatised tooth is then fixed to the wire in the same fashion.

After the procedure, the patient should be warned of the guarded/poor prognosis of the tooth. They should attend their GDP as an emergency as soon as possible so formal vitality assessment and a long-term treatment plan can be undertaken.

TOP TIPS

- It is important to remember that these procedures are often carried out in the ED where there is limited dental equipment.
- Unlike in a dental clinic, there is often no suction available. Also, there is often no assistant. Therefore preparation is key, as this procedure is technically challenging.

SUTURING OF THE FACE AND MOUTH

The principles of suturing the face are no different to suturing elsewhere on the body. Where possible, wounds should undergo layered closure, with non-dissolvable sutures applied to the skin. This allows the surgeon to dictate when sutures should be removed depending on different healing rates for different parts of the face. In addition bites should be of equal size and depth. Knots should be tightly secured, and placed to one side of the suture line. Wound edges require eversion to maximise healing.

The table below highlights what sutures should be used superficially on various areas, although often the choice of suture is dependent on surgeon preference and, often, local stock. In young children (for whom suture removal in the clinic could be an emotionally traumatic procedure) it is advisable to use a rapidly dissolving suture (Vicryl™ rapide) on the skin instead of non-resorbable materials. This way, the externalised suture knots can be 'rubbed off' at day 5 with a damp flannel by the parent(s).

Table 5.2: Appropriate suture, suture size and time of suture removal for various facial areas

Area	Suture	Size	Stitch	ROS
Lip (Vermillion)	Vicryl™ rapide	5/0 or 6/0	Interrupted with buried knot	N/A
Lip (Vermillion Border)	Ethilon™	5/0	Interrupted stitch	5 days
Eyelid	Ethilon™	6/0	Subcuticular continuous with ends left long to facilitate removal. Alternatively, interrupted sutures can be used (but with caution as to avoid causing an ectropion).	3-5 days
Ala	Ethilon™	6/0	Interrupted	5-7 days
Pinna	Ethilon™	6/0	Interrupted	7 days
Cheeks, Chin and Forehead	Ethilon™	5/0	Interrupted	5 days
Intraoral	Vicryl™ rapide	3/0 or 4/0	Interrupted	N/A
Deep dermal/ fascial tension sutures.	Vicryl™	3/0 or 4/0	Interrupted with buried knot	N/A

PROCEDURES

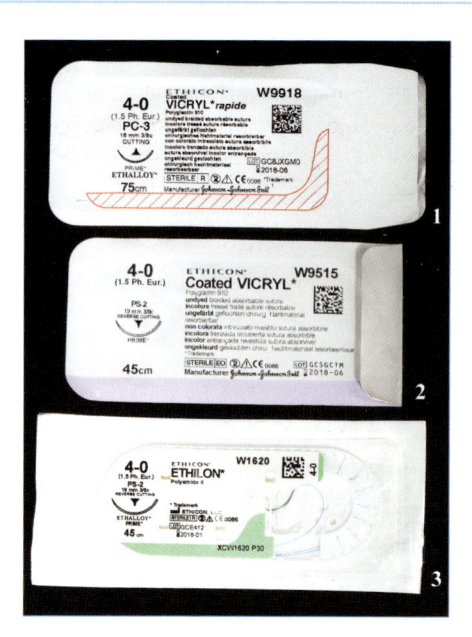

Fig 5.14. Examples of suture material (in packaging)

1. 4/0 Vicryl™ rapide
2. 4/0 Vicryl™
3. 4/0 Ethilon™

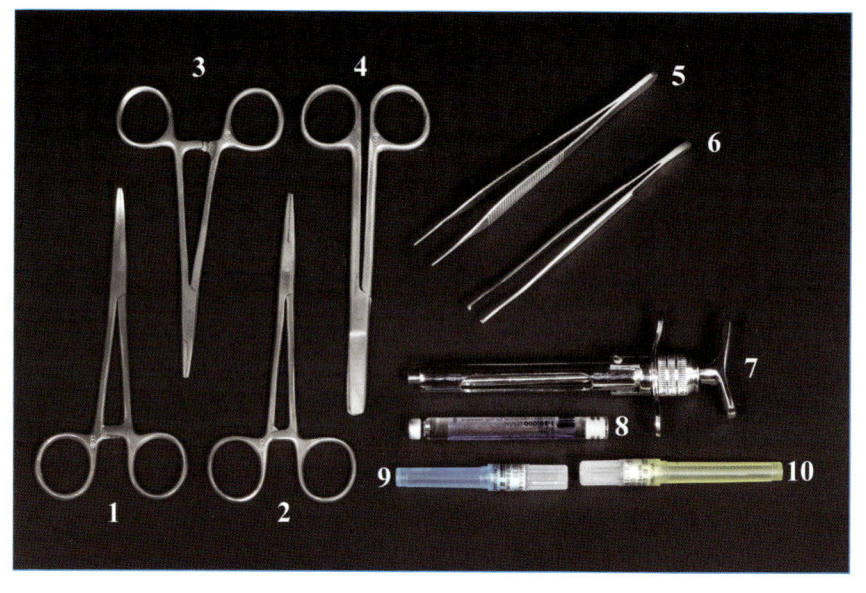

Fig 5.15. Surgical instruments used during facial laceration wound closure

1. Curved Spencer Wells forceps
2. Straight Spencer Wells forceps
3. Needle holding forceps
4. Suture cutting scissors
5. Anatomical (non-toothed) forceps
6. Gillies (toothed) forceps
7. Dental syringe
8. LA cartridge
9. Short dental needle (25mm)
10. Long dental needle (35mm)

WOUND CLOSURE

In this section we provide a step-by-step approach to closing facial lacerations, together with a detailed discussion of a few facial areas that often cause difficulty.

1. Obtain informed consent. Often verbal consent is satisfactory for closure of minor wounds but the patient should be warned of all possible risks including bleeding, infection, scarring, neurovascular injury and need for further treatment such as wound debridement/dressings etc. Consider using a consent form if the injury is extensive.

2. Anaesthetise the wound. This can be done either with local infiltration along the wound margins or a regional block. Local infiltration is acceptable for small wounds, but with larger more complex wounds a regional block is preferred as it reduces the tissue distorting effects of injecting the LA (for choice of LA see 'Local anaesthetic' page 160).

3. Prepare the wound. Using Betadine®/Chlorhexidine and where possible, create a sterile operative area with sterile paper/linen drapes.

4. Explore the wound. Look for neurovascular and other structures such as ducts and muscle belly/tendon. Are they visible? Are they intact? If in doubt, discuss with the on-call senior for definitive exploration and repair.

5. Radiography? If you are unsure of the possibility of foreign bodies in the soft tissues, a soft tissue radiograph can be useful. However, this investigation will only show radiopaque foreign bodies. Therefore some glasses, wood or plastic may not be identifiable; hence the importance of thorough wound exploration.

6. Irrigate the wound thoroughly with copious volumes of normal saline. If you are happy in achieving adequate decontamination with irrigation, proceed to closure. For injuries where significant contamination has occurred, consider debridement and wound closure under GA (see page 62). Debris not removed can present months afterwards as a pigmented/tattooed area, which is very difficult to manage non-surgically.

7. Closure. Layered subcutaneous and dermal suturing is required to ensure a tension-free repair at the skin surface. Often this is best achieved by using as fine a suture material as possible but with multiple suture points giving overall strength to the repair but minimising the tissue inflammatory response and subsequent scarring. Superficial sutures can then be placed. (For the choice of suture technique and suture material, see Table 5.2 above.)

SPECIFIC AREAS – THE LIP

If you are happy to proceed with closure of a lip laceration crossing the vermillion border, it is common practice to use a non-absorbable suture on the skin (e.g. 6/0 nylon) and then convert to a rapidly absorbable suture (e.g. 6/0 Vicryl™ rapide) for the vermillion and mucosa as this does not require suture removal (which can be particularly painful, and difficult in the case of rapidly epithelializing mucosal surfaces). Any continuation of suturing intraorally should be with a similar absorbable suture but thicker gauges (e.g. 4/0) can be used, as there is less of an aesthetic concern.

If the laceration is a 'through-and-through' laceration (i.e. dividing the lip through all tissue layers) or partial thickness but involving orbicularis muscle, the muscle should be re-apposed with strong interrupted sutures (Fig 5.16). For this, a slowly dissolvable suture such as Vicryl™ or PDS™ of 3/0 or 4/0 gauge would be sufficient.

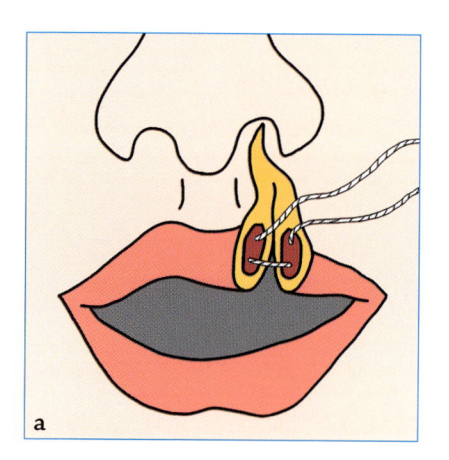

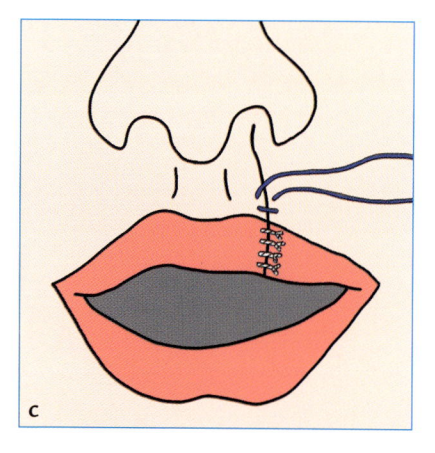

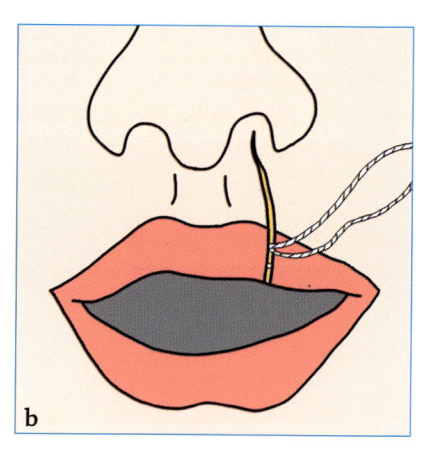

Fig 5.16. Suturing a full thickness laceration of the upper lip that crosses the vermillion border

   a) *Closure is in layers, beginning with the muscular layer.*
   b) *Continue to the subcutaneous layer. This should oppose the wound edge nicely.*
   c) *Finally close the skin, vermillion and mucosa with superficial interrupted sutures.*

TOP TIPS
- When suturing intraorally, it is best to begin the suture at the mobile mucosa and stitch towards the more stable mucosa. This will minimise the risk of 'cheese-wiring' through the wound edges.
- When tying a knot intraorally, ensure the free end of the suture is short as this allows easier control during knot-tying.
- Take great care to safely control your needle during suturing and knot tying, especially near the patient's eyes.

BRIDLE WIRING

In mandibular fractures, patients can suffer considerable pain and discomfort due to the mobile bone edges moving against one and other, and also bleeding from the fracture site. As such, in fractures of the body, parasymphysis and symphysis, as a temporary measure, wire can be used to fix the two edges together.

FIG 5.17. BRIDLE WIRING PROCEDURE FOR A MANDIBULAR SYMPHYSEAL FRACTURE.

a) Administer LA and relocate the two edges of bone as best you can.
b) A 0.35mm/0.45mm diameter wire is loaded into a heavy artery clip. This wire is passed around the second nearest tooth not involved in the fracture site, buccal to lingual in the inter-proximal space above the gingival papilla.
c) The wire is grasped on the lingual side and reversed, then passed lingual to buccal, in the same inter-proximal position, around the second tooth from the fracture site on the opposite side of the fracture.
d) The two wire ends are united to form a loop of wire and cut to equal length.
e) The wire ends are then wound together in a clockwise fashion.
f) To tighten the wires, grip the wire end with the forceps and rotate the wrist while loosely holding the forceps.
g) The free end of wire is cut approximately 1cm in length.
h) This free end is then curved around into the inter-dental area to avoid mucosal trauma.

ON-CALL IN ORAL AND MAXILLOFACIAL SURGERY   179

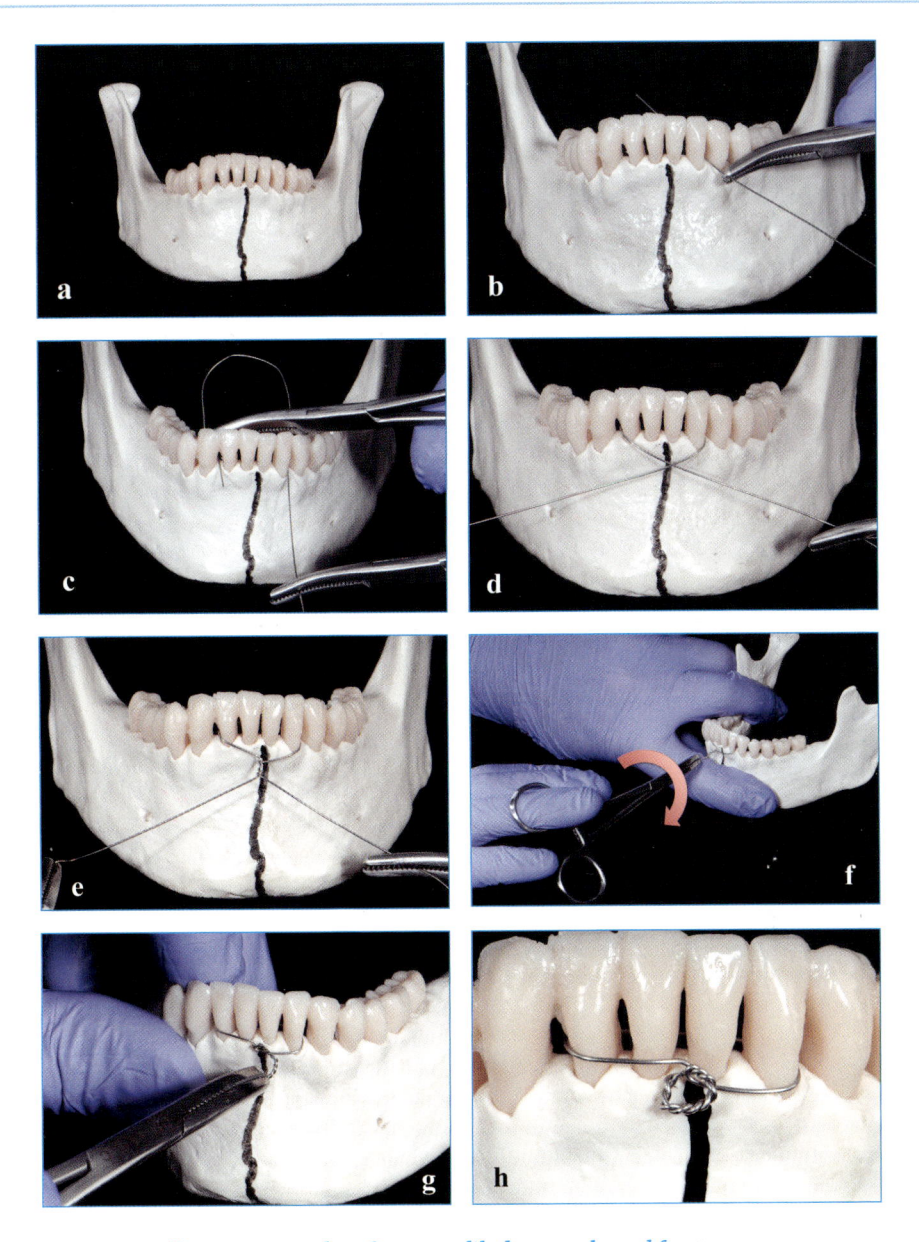

Fig 5.17. Bridle wiring procedure for a mandibular symphyseal fracture

PROCEDURES

NASAL PACKING

ANTERIOR NASAL PACKING

The procedure below describes the insertion of a nasal tampon (Merocel®) or an intranasal balloon (Rapid Rhino®). However, other methods are available.

1. Ensure a suitable length nasal tampon/balloon is used (i.e. to ensure that it is long enough to compress the bleeding site).
2. Explain to the patient what is involved and gain consent.
3. Only if the patient is not in extremis, consider applying some local anaesthetic spray to the nasal cavity bilaterally.
4. Lubricate the tampon/balloon with a water-based lubricant (KY® Jelly) or antibiotic ointment (e.g. Naseptin® or Chloramphenicol).
5. Insert the tampon/balloon (horizontally) along the floor of the nasal cavity to its entire length.
6. To aid rapid expansion of the nasal tampon, syringe a small amount of normal saline (using a syringe with flexible plastic cannula tip) alongside the tampon. With the intranasal balloon use an air-filled 10ml syringe to inflate the device.

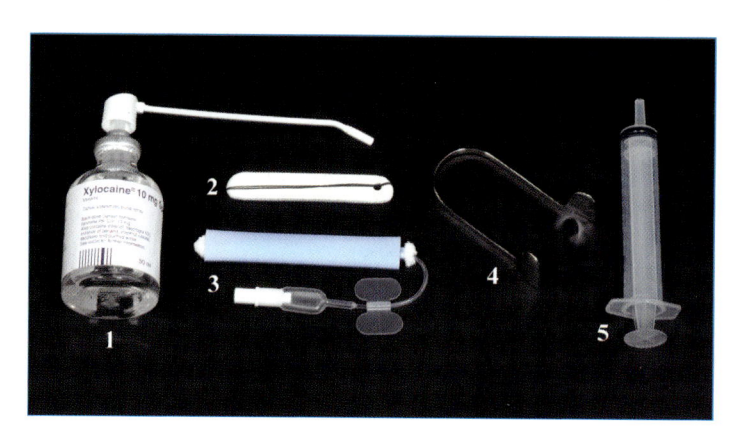

Fig 5.18. Anterior nasal packs and equipment for nasal packing

1. *Nasal anaesthetic spray*
2. *Merocel® nasal tampon*
3. *Rapid Rhino® intranasal balloon*
4. *Nasal speculum*
5. *10ml syringe to inflate intranasal tampon*

7. Secure the tampon/balloon cords to the face with adhesive tape (e.g. zinc-oxide tape).
8. Assess the effectiveness of your packing. Consider inserting another tampon/balloon contralaterally to increase pressure on the ipsilateral side. If the patient continues to bleed, consider using a posterior or combined (posteroanterior) packing technique instead.

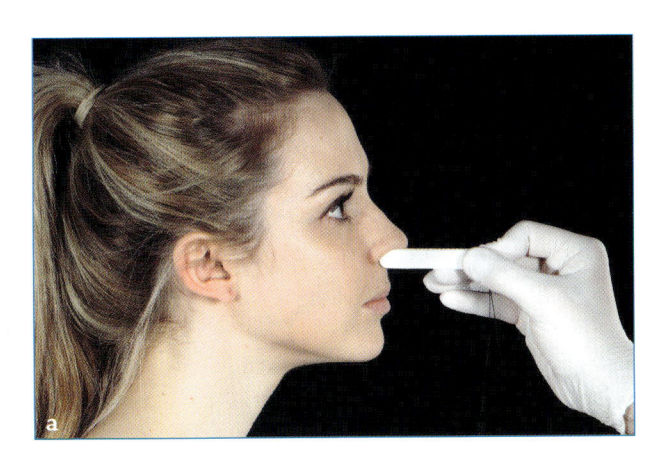

Fig 5.19. Procedure for anterior nasal packing using a Merocel® nasal tampon. (a) Insertion of the tampon (note the angle of insertion) and (b) the tampon expanded within the nasal cavity.

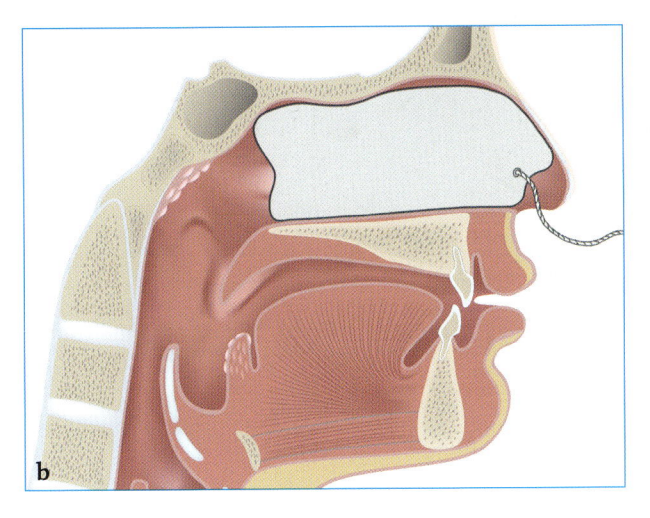

POSTERIOR NASAL PACKING

The procedure below describes the use of one or two Foley catheters to achieve posterior haemostasis. Other methods are available.

1. Explain to the patient what is involved and gain consent (not possible if the patient is unconscious)
2. Only if the patient is not in extremis, consider applying some local anaesthetic spray to the nostrils.
3. Lubricate the catheter with a water-based lubricant (KY® Jelly) or antibiotic ointment (e.g. Naseptin® or Chloramphenicol).
4. Inflate and deflate the catheter balloon with an air-filled syringe to check for any leaks. Most catheter balloons inflate to 10ml volume but check the inflation port/catheter packaging for the appropriate volume.
5. Insert the catheter into the nostril with most bleeding. Pass the catheter along the entirety of the floor of the nasal cavity, inflate the catheter balloon and gently pull the catheter to ensure that it sits firmly against the posterior nasal aperture. The tip of the catheter may just be visible intraorally before inflation.
6. Commonly, a second catheter is required to control posterior haemorrhage. This is placed in the contralateral nostril so that the patient is packed bilaterally (you may need to deflate the original catheter balloon again to pass the second catheter, then re-inflate both of them simultaneously).
7. Having packed the postnasal space with catheter balloon(s), maintain anterior tension on the catheters whilst simultaneously packing anteriorly to the catheter with a lubricated nasal tampon/balloon (see 'Anterior nasal packing' above) or with BIPP ribbon gauze.
8. Finally, with continuing gentle but firm tension on the Foley catheter(s), place a protective gauze dressing over the columella and alar rim (as to prevent pressure necrosis), and clamp the catheter(s) in place with a plastic umbilical clip or artery clip. If a clip is not easily available, the ends of two catheters can be tied together over the protective gauze padding to produce the same effect. It is essential to maintain tension on the catheters to provide a haemostatic/pressure effect on the postnasal space/posterior nasal aperture.

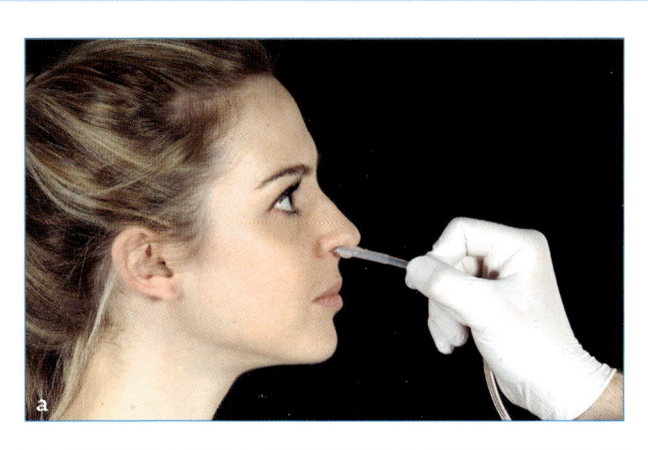

Fig 5.20. Procedure for posterior nasal packing using a Foley catheter. (a) Insertion of the catheter (note the angle of insertion) and (b) the catheter balloon expanded within the posterior nasal space.

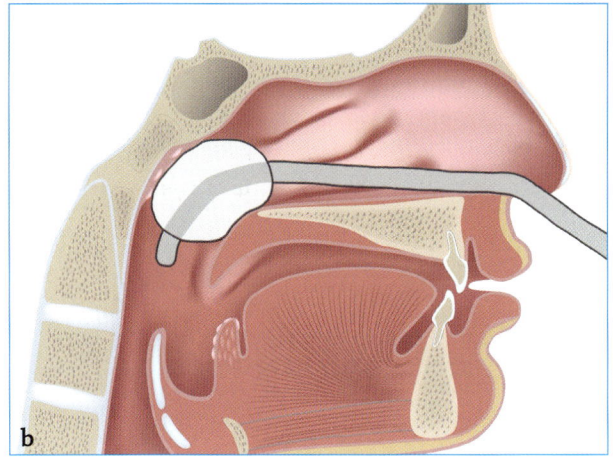

DRAINING ABSCESSES UNDER LOCAL ANAESTHETIC

SKIN ABSCESS/INFECTED SEBACEOUS CYST

As with all abscesses, treatment involves drainage of the accumulated pus with healing by secondary intention, once the areas of infection have resolved. While this is a simple procedure, you should always be mindful of scar formation and the underlying anatomical structures:

Where possible, incisions should be placed in line with relaxed skin tension lines of the face, to aid cosmesis. Be aware of the facial nerve and its branches within the face. Notably the marginal mandibular branch situated under the lower border of the mandible.

1. Anaesthetise the area. A regional block is preferable as anaesthesia is more likely to be effective in this situation than local infiltration. However, either/both can be used.
2. Using a size 11 blade make a small incision over the swelling piercing the abscess cavity.
3. Thoroughly 'milk' out the pus.
4. Using a syringe, irrigate the cavity with normal saline.
5. If you have optimal anaesthesia, grasp a piece of gauze in the tips of a pair of forceps and in a scraping fashion clean the inside of the cavity.
6. Consider placing a glove drain to aid drainage.
7. Discharge the patient on oral antibiotics and review in clinic (or GP/GDP) in approximately 1 week.

BUCCAL SULCUS ABSCESS

As previously discussed, those patients presenting with a superficial localised dental abscess, usually an intraoral collection in the buccal sulcus, with no systemic compromise, are amenable to drainage under LA in the ED and discharge with oral antibiotics.

1. Anaesthetise the area. Preferably a regional block, local infiltration to the overlying mucosa, and/or by spraying the affected region with ethyl chloride. LA may be less effective in the presence of infection so ethyl chloride may be a suitable adjunct or alternative.
2. Identify and palpate the area of maximum fluctuance.
3. Using a size 11 blade make a small incision into the mucosa overlying the area of maximum fluctuance, making sure to extend down to bone.
4. Milk out the pus and irrigate the cavity with normal saline.
5. A drain may be useful (e.g. glove drain or Yates drain) and can be placed within the abscess cavity, especially in the mandible due to lack of gravitational drainage.
6. Discharge the patient on oral antibiotics and review in clinic (or GDP) in approximately 1 week.

PINNA HAEMATOMA

A pinna haematoma classically presents soon after blunt trauma (e.g. a punch) to the external ear (auricle/pinna). The skin overlying the cartilage of the pinna is thin and disturbance of the subdermal blood supply risks vascularity of the skin, particularly when compressed by an underlying haematoma. This puts the skin at risk of necrosis and a potential risk of developing a serious soft tissue infection/chondritis of the pinna. In addition, a large haematoma in the long term may cause significant fibrosis of both the skin and underlying cartilage, resulting in an unsightly 'cauliflower ear' deformity. Consequently, in the presence of a pinna haematoma, drainage should be performed as promptly as possible.

1. The procedure is most commonly performed under local anaesthesia in the ED using a ring-block technique to anaesthetise the auricle (Fig 5.11).
2. Under sterile conditions (Chlorhexidine/Tisept/Betadine® prep and drapes where possible), the skin over the most convex part of the haematoma swelling is incised with a small (3-4mm) stab incision using a size 11 blade (this may need to be repeated on the medial aspect of the pinna if there is swelling superficial to the cartilage there as well).
3. The haematoma is 'milked' from the swelling and the cavity gently irrigated using a syringe of saline and plastic IV cannula tip (18G).
4. Apply a non-adherent dressing to the incision site(s) (e.g. Mepitel®/Jelonet®). Overlying this a sterile cotton wool roll is placed (on the lateral and medial surface of the pinna, directly overlying the haematoma site).
5. Finally, place a single 4/0 or 5/0 nylon suture through the dental rolls/gauze/dressings/pinna, from one side to the other, and pass the needle back through again. Tie the suture down securely with the aim of compressing the wound sites with the overlying dressings, to prevent reformation of the haematoma (Fig 5.21).
6. Arrange for the patient to be seen in the outpatient clinic in 3-5 days for removal of the sutured dressing.

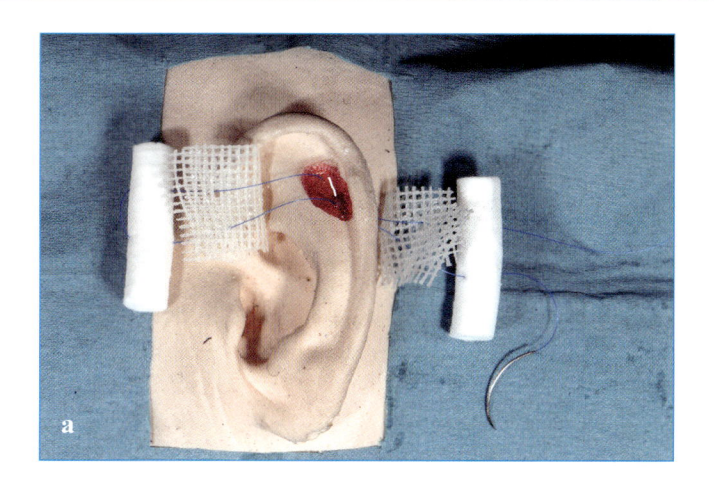

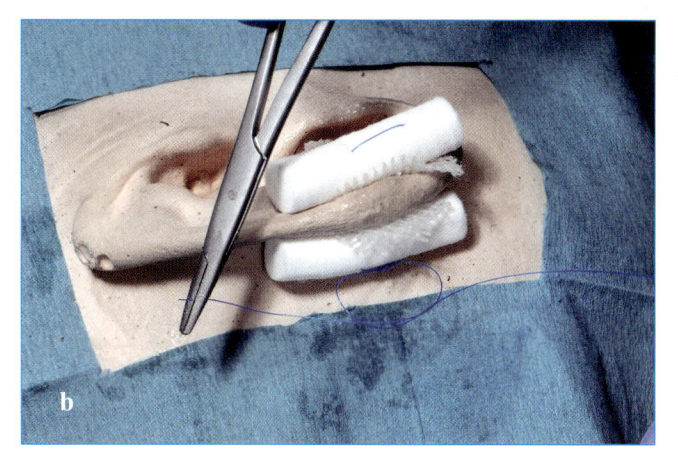

Fig 5.21. Procedure for draining and dressing a pinna haematoma
a) *Pinna haematoma of left ear. Incision made (white line) and haematoma drained. Cotton wool rolls, and non-adherent dressing sutured in place.*
b) *Suture is tightened. Dressing lies as shown.*

SEPTAL HAEMATOMA

A haematoma of the septum of the nose is fairly uncommon but may occur following nasal trauma or surgery (manipulation of nasal bone fractures or septo-rhinoplasty for example). On examination, it will typically present as a visible boggy swelling overlying the cartilage septum (but may extend further posteriorly). The cartilage of the septum derives its blood supply from the perichondrium on both sides. Therefore in theory, a compressing (typically subperichondrial) haematoma may precipitate avascular necrosis of the cartilage. Therefore, as in the case of a pinna haematoma, this should be drained as soon as possible.

1. Clean the haematoma site with a damp gauze swab soaked in saline/prep solution.
2. Make a small (3-4mm) incision over the most convex part of the boggy swelling with a size 11 blade.
3. Place a fine-bore sucker over the incision and apply pressure with a digit in the contralateral nostril to 'milk' the haematoma from the cavity.
4. Then either:
    a. Pack both nostrils anteriorly to gently but effectively compress the septum and prevent recurrence of a haematoma (see 'Anterior nasal packing' page 180).
    b. Place a quilting suture using 5/0 Vicryl™ rapide (several passes through the mucoperichondrium and cartilaginous septum) to reduce the potential space where haematoma could otherwise recollect.

The patient should be reviewed in clinic. If packs were placed, these should ideally be removed at 24-48 hours and a wound check should be performed at 1-2 weeks regardless.

FLEXIBLE NASOENDOSCOPY

Flexible nasoendoscopy is a chairside examination that allows visualisation of the posterior nasal cavity, the nasopharynx, the hypopharynx and the larynx (Fig 1.8). It can be useful in a number of situations. These include recurrent epistaxis, persistent dysphagia, suspected malignancy and foreign body inhalation. It may also provide valuable information about the condition of the airway in neck space infections.

The procedure can be carried out with the following method, although techniques vary:

1. The patient should be sat upright with their head supported with a head rest.
2. Nasal anaesthetic spray should be sprayed into each nostril. This may take up to 5 minutes to take effect.
3. The flexible nasoendoscope (Fig 5.22) should be connected to the light source.
4. The tip of the scope is held with the non-dominant hand and the control head operated with the dominant hand.
5. The camera is controlled using the lever on the control head, usually with the thumb or index finger. The camera head moves approximately 90 degrees in the vertical plane only.
6. The correct camera-control head orientation can be checked by looking through the lens, typically at the writing on a pack of white gauze.
7. Lubricating jelly can be added around the tip of the scope although the camera tip should be avoided.
8. Nostril patency can be checked to assess which side is more patent.
9. The tip of the scope is passed through the nostril and advanced horizontally along the floor of the nose.
10. When the scope reaches the posterior pharyngeal wall (Fig 5.23a), the tip can be angled downwards which should allow continued advancement towards the larynx (Fig 5.23b).
11. Once visualised, symmetrical vocal cord movement can also be assessed by asking the patient to say 'eeee'.
12. If assessing patients for a possible oropharyngeal malignancy, they should be prompted to stick their tongue out which will allow you to visualise the base of tongue and vallecula more adequately.
13. The scope can then be removed, disinfected and stored.

The following information should be documented in the patient's case notes:
- Local anaesthetic used.
- Ease and site of scope entry.
- Presence of pathology in/at: nasal cavity, tongue base, vallecula, piriform fossae, epiglottis, arytenoid cartilages.
- The amount and symmetry of vocal cord movement should also be documented, as should any swellings or oedema of the vocal cords.

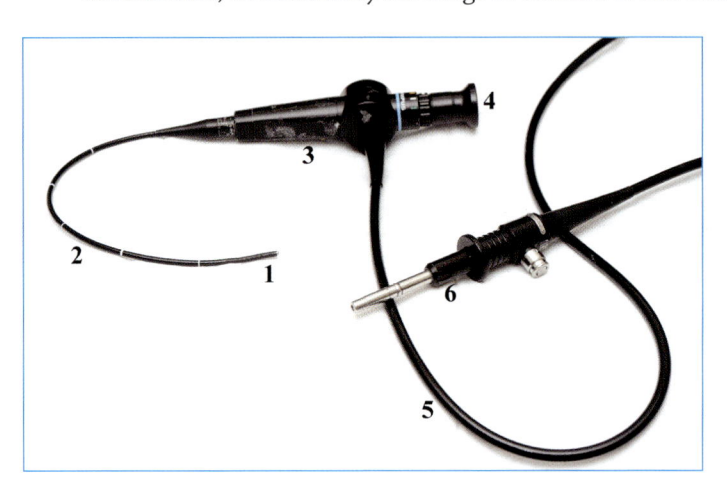

Fig 5.22. Flexible nasoendoscope

1. *Manoeuvrable tip*
2. *Insertion tube*
3. *Control head with angulation control lever*
4. *Eyepiece (or attachment for camera head)*
5. *Universal cord/'umbilical' cable*
6. *Light connector section (to attach to light source)*

ON-CALL IN ORAL AND MAXILLOFACIAL SURGERY   191

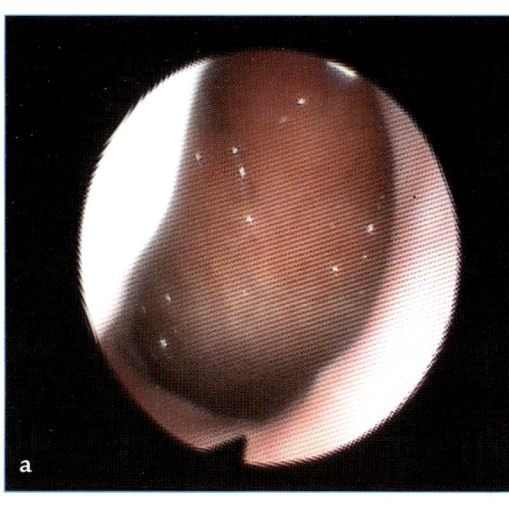

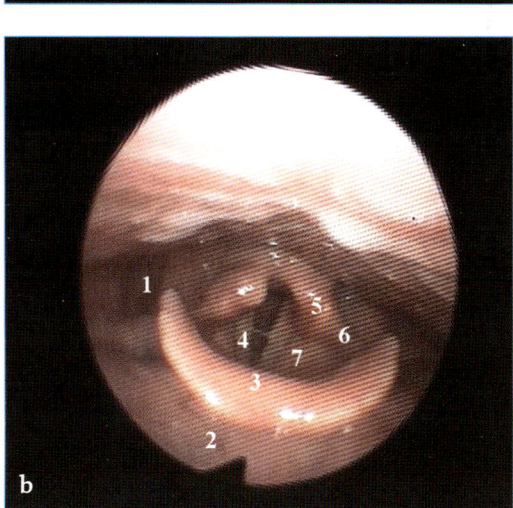

Fig 5.23. Flexible nasoendoscope images

a) *Within nasal cavity, viewing posterior nasal space*
b) *View down into larynx*
1. Piriform fossa
2. Base of tongue
3. Epiglottis
4. Vocal cord
5. Arytenoid cartilage
6. Aryepiglottic fold
7. Vestibular fold

PROCEDURES

TOP TIPS

- Silicone spray can help avoid fogging of the lens.
- If fogging occurs, the lens can be gently touched against the mucosa or tongue to clean it.
- On insertion, staying below the inferior turbinate ensures correct placement.
- Swallowing, blowing out the cheeks and the Valsalva manoeuvres can all be used to facilitate advancement of the scope and improve the anatomical view.

LATERAL CANTHOTOMY

A lateral canthotomy is a procedure carried out to relieve the increased pressure that occurs in orbital compartment syndrome, to alleviate the effects of a retrobulbar haemorrhage. While it may be unlikely that you are expected to carry out this procedure unaided, in an emergency situation it may make the difference in saving the sight of a patient's eye.

This procedure involves dividing the lateral canthus of the eye down to the orbital rim (canthotomy) as well the option to release the inferior and or superior crus of the lateral canthal tendon (cantholysis) (Fig 5.24a).

1. The area involved (namely the upper lateral aspect of the face and eye) should be prepped and draped.
2. LA (lidocaine with adrenaline) should be injected into the lateral canthus.
3. Position a clamp with the tips on either side of the lateral canthus (at the lateral corner of the eye) and advance until the tips touch the bony orbit.
4. Clamp for 30 seconds.
5. Cut through the crushed demarcated line using sharp scissors, all the way to the orbital rim (Fig 5.24b).
6. You may or may not see an escape of blood once this is completed.

A further cantholysis procedure can be done in addition to further alleviate pressure:

1. The lower eyelid is grasped with forceps and can now be pulled downwards.
2. The inferior crus of the canthal tendon can now be seen or palpated.
3. This is then cut again using sharp scissors (Fig 5.24c).
4. The orbit can be re-assessed and the upper crus of the canthal tendon can also be cut if necessary.

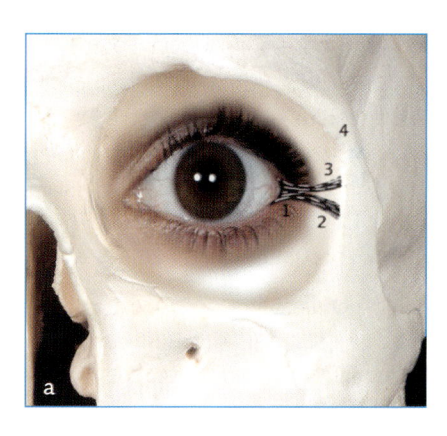

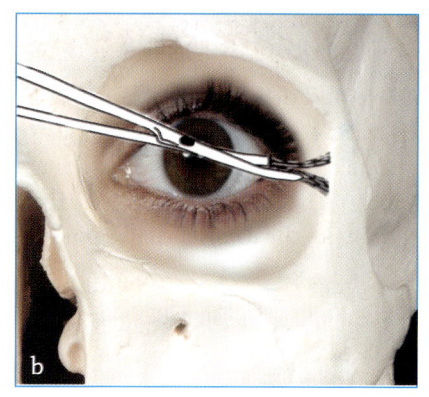

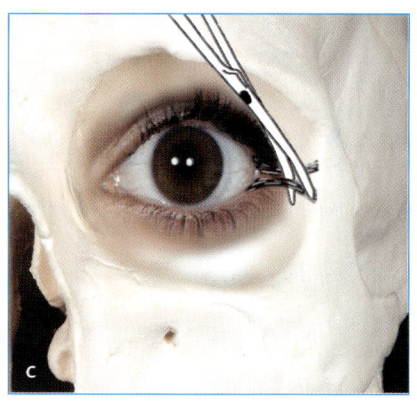

Fig 5.24. Left eye superimposed over orbital skeleton, to show anatomy and incision for lateral canthotomy and inferior cantholysis

  a) *1 – Lateral cathal tendon, 2 – Inferior crus of canthal tendon, 3 – Superior crus of canthal tendon, 4 – Orbital rim*
  b) *Cutting the lateral canthus with sharp scissors (lateral canthotomy)*
  c) *Inferior crus of the canthal tendon can also be cut (inferior cantholysis)*

INDEX

A

Acute closed lock (see Anchored disc)
Acute necrotizing ulcerative gingivitis 87
Acute orbital compartment syndrome 57
Adenoid cystic carcinoma 120
Admissions 5
Airway
- management 45-46, 86, 97-99
- obstruction (signs) 82
Alveolar Osteitis (see Dry socket)
Alvogyl® 71
Analgesia 37
Anatomy
- Tooth 12
- Oral and nasal cavity 22-23
- Pharynx 23
- Nerves 24
- Neck 25-31, 77
- Facial 19-21
Anchored disc phenomenon 114
Antibiotics 38, 52, 80
Antiemetics 38
Apthous ulcers 125-126
Arthrocentesis 135
Arthroscopy 135
Articaine 161
Atypical facial pain 137
Auscultation sites 11
Avulsion injury (of tooth) 72

B

Basal cell carcinoma (BCC) 122
Bimaxillary osteotomy (consent) 147
Bite blocks 46
Bleeding gums 87
Bleeding socket 69-70
Blood cultures 158
Blood tests 47,
Bridle wiring 46, 178-179
Buccal abscess 185
Buccal space 77
Bupivicaine 161
Burning mouth syndrome 137

Burns, facial 65-66
Buttresses (facial) 48

C

Cancer 115-119, 130-132
Candidiasis 129-130
Cannulation, IV 156-157
Cerebrospinal Fluid (CSF) 45
Class 1/2/3 (dental occlusion) 17-18
Clerking 7-11
Computed Tomography (CT, radiology) 33, 36, 86
Concussion (of tooth) 72
Condylar fracture (unilateral) 111
Consent 142-150
Crossbite 17

D

Dermatofibroma 122
Deciduous dentition 14-15
Dental abscess (see orofacial and neck space infection)
Dental extraction (consent) 148
Dentoalveolar fracture 50
Discharge summary 5
DPT (OPG, radiology) 32, 34
Drug charts 138
Dry socket 71

E

Epistaxis 67-68, 182
Eruption dates 16
Examination
- Cardiovascular 9
- Respiratory 9
- Abdominal 9
- Neurological 10
- Facial 41-45, 48
Extrusion injury (of tooth) 72
Eye movements 42
Eye signs 51

F

Facial
-Infection 77-82, 84, 184-185
-Trauma 41-45
-Lacerations 61-64, 175
-Anatomy (see Anatomy, Facial)

-Examination (see Examination, Facial)
FDI system 15
Feeding, enteral 103-105
Fibroma 128
Flaps 100-102
- assessment 101
- classification 100
- monitoring 101
- failure 102
Flexible nasoendoscopy 189-191
Foley catheter 183
Frey's syndrome 121
G
Glasgow coma scale (GCS) 59-60
Glucose control
- pre-operative management 95-96
- sliding scale 96
H
Haemangioma 122
Hess chart 112-113
History 7
- in trauma 41
House-Brackmann scale 121
I
ID block (see Inferior alveolar nerve block)
Inferior alveolar nerve block 161-166
Infra-orbital nerve block 167
Inpatient lists 5
Instruments (surgical) 39-40
Intra-oral malignancy 131-132
Intravenous fluids 89-93
Intrusion injury (of tooth) 72
K
Keratocanthoma 122
L
Lateral canthotomy 192-193
Lateral cephalogram (radiology) 32
Lateral luxation injury (of tooth) 72
Lateral oblique (radiology) 33
Le Fort fracture
- classification 49
- management of 54
Lentigo maligna 123
Lichen planus 126-128
Lichenoid reaction 126-128
Lidocaine 161
Lip wound closure 176-177
Local anaesthetic 160

Ludwigs angina 82
Lymph node levels (of the neck) 29-31
M
Magnetic Resonance Imaging (MRI, radiology) 33
Malignant melanoma 123
Mandibular fracture 55-56
- consent 144
Meibomian cyst 123
Mental nerve block 166
Merocel® nasal tampon 180-181
MRSA 139
Mucocoele 128-129
Multidisciplinary team (MDT) 115
Myofascial pain 135
N
Naevus 123
Nasal bone fracture 52
- consent 145
Naso-orbito-ethmoidal complex fracture 53
Nasal packing
-anterior 180-181
-posterior 182-183
Nasogastric (NG) tube 103-104
Nasojejunal (NJ) tube 103-104
Neck
-anatomy (see anatomy)
-lymph node levels (see lymph node levels)
-trauma zones (see trauma zones)
Neck dissection (consent) 150
Necrotising fasciitis 81
Nerve supply (sensory) of face 23-25
Non-healing ulcer 130
O
Occipitomental view (radiology) 32, 35-36
Occlusal radiograph 32
Occlusion (dental) 17
Occulocardiac reflex 51
Open bite 17
Operating list 141
OPG (DPT, radiology) 32, 34
Oral candidiasis 129-130
Orbital cellulitis 80
Orbital floor fracture 50
- review in clinic 112
- consent 147

Orofacial and neck space infections 77
- consent for drainage 145
Overbite 17
Overjet 17

P

Pain
- history 7
- relief (see analgesia)
Palliative care 118
Parotidectomy (consent) 150
Patient assessment 7-11, 106-109
Percutaneous endoscopic gastrostomy (PEG) tube 103, 104
Pinna haematoma 185-187
Pleomorphic adenoma 120
Post extraction bleeding (see bleeding socket)
Posteroanterior (PA) view of mandible (radiology) 33, 34
Pre-assessment 138-141
Prilocaine 161
Pupillary responses 42

R

Rapid Rhino® intranasal balloon 180
Recurrent aphthous ulceration 125-126
Refeeding syndrome 105
Referrals 3-4
Retrobulbar haemorrhage 51, 57-58,
Ring block of external ear 169

S

Salivary gland 119-121
Scalpel blades 40
Sebaceous cyst 84, 184
Sebhorrhoeic keratosis 123
Septal haematoma 188
Skin lesions 122-124
Shock 107
Sialadenitis, acute 83
Sialolithiasis 119
Skin tags 123
Sliding scale (see glucose management)
Snellen chart 43
Solar keratosis 124

Splinting 170-172
Squamous cell carcinoma (SCC)
- skin 124
- oral cavity 130-132
- salivary gland 120
Sublingual space 77
Subluxation injury (of tooth) 72
Submandibular space 77
Submentovertex view (radiology) 32, 35
Supraorbital nerve block 168-169
Supratrochlear nerve block 168-169
Surgical blades 40
Surgicel® 69-70
Suturing material 173-175

T

Tetanus 63
TMJ
- anchored disc 114
- assessment of 133-134
- disorders 134-135
- dislocation 75-76
Tracheostomy 97-99
-consent 149
Trauma zones (of the neck) 28-29, 85-86
Triangles (of the neck) 26-28
Trigeminal neuralgia 137-138

U

Ultrasound scan (radiology) 33
Ulcer, non-healing 130

V

Venupuncture 155-156
Vitamin K 109

W

Warfarin management 109-110
White-eyed blowout fracture 51
WHO pain ladder 37
Wound closure 175

Z

Zsigmondy-Palmar system 14
Zygomatic fracture 53
- review in clinic 113
- consent 146

NOTES

NOTES